THIS BOOK IS TO BE RETURNED ON OR BEFORE THE LAST DATE STAMPED BELOW

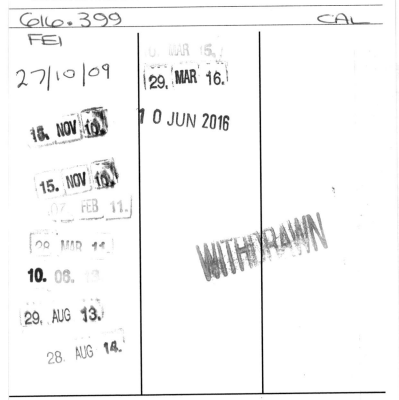

Overcoming Common Problems Series

Selected titles

A full list of titles is available from Sheldon Press,
36 Causton Street, London SW1P 4ST and on our website at
www.sheldonpress.co.uk

Overcoming Common Problems Series

Overcoming Common Problems Series

Overcoming Common Problems

Living with Gluten Intolerance

JANE FEINMANN

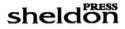

First published in Great Britain in 2009

Sheldon Press
36 Causton Street
London SW1P 4ST

British Library Cataloguing-in-Publication Data
A catalogue record for this book is available from the British Library

ISBN 978-1-84709-057-7

1 3 5 7 9 10 8 6 4 2

Typeset by Fakenham Photosetting Ltd, Fakenham, Norfolk
Printed in Great Britain by Ashford Colour Press

Produced on paper from sustainable forests

For Mary

Contents

Note to the reader

This is not a medical book and is not intended to replace advice from your doctor. Consult your pharmacist or doctor if you believe you have any of the symptoms described, and if you think you might need medical help.

Introduction

With 195,000 edible plants in the world, the modern diet is very exclusive. With this vast range of potential plants to choose from, just two or three provide 50 per cent of the calories in today's typical diet. The main staple is wheat, with a little rye and barley thrown in – all cereals that are edible only when cooked, or more commonly baked. What makes them such a success is a sticky protein called gluten.

This wonder ingredient – the part of the grain that makes bread rise and creates its light, doughy texture, as well as creating food that is both chewy and absorbent – is responsible for some of the most delicious, nutritious and easy to prepare foods in our diet: bread, cakes and biscuits as well as pasta, pizza and pies.

Yet for a minority of people, gluten causes problems. For well over half a century it has been known to cause the major digestive disorder coeliac disease – a health problem that triggers unpleasant and potentially dangerous symptoms.

More recently, there have been many anecdotal claims, underpinned by some scientific evidence, that a far larger group of people may have problems with gluten. As many as one in eight of us could have problems digesting gluten, causing the same kind of symptoms as coeliac disease, and perhaps overlapping with other digestive disorders such as *Candida* infection and irritable bowel syndrome (IBS).

A growing number of people believe that they are intolerant to gluten. An even larger number believe that cutting down on gluten-containing food is good for their health, in the same way as it is a healthy choice to cut back on saturated fat or increase the amount of fruit and vegetables in the diet. This new trend has changed our shopping habits and our expectations of caterers in local cafés and gourmet restaurants alike. Yet there is a significant difference in this choice compared with low-fat milk or going vegetarian. Gluten intolerance is still highly controversial, and anyone making a choice to cut back on gluten or stop eating it altogether is unlikely to have the support of doctors or indeed friends and family.

If you decide to buy more fruit and vegetables or to switch to semi-skimmed milk then you'll get nothing but praise, but if you let people know that you're cutting back on gluten, or worse cutting out gluten, then you should expect a reaction that may be nothing short of derision.

The medical profession has long been sceptical about the existence of food intolerance generally, and there is little sign of a change. Here's Dr Clare Gerada of the Royal College of General Practitioners, dismissing the problem in January 2008 as 'just tosh'. Patients who claim to have a food intolerance, she says, are simply preoccupied with what they eat.

> It becomes central to their lives and that is a giveaway that the real cause of the problem is less likely to be a rogue sensitivity to pannacotta but more likely to derive from a disliked job or a marriage in turmoil or the beginning of a breakdown, misery which is manifesting itself as an upset tummy or a regular headache.

Other doctors express even more concern about the dangers of giving up gluten, with highly respected experts regularly dismissing gluten intolerance as a 'celebrity-endorsed faddy diet' that can 'set women on the slippery slope towards an eating disorder'.

And if doctors are unsympathetic, public figures can be even more unkind. Laughing at food intolerance has become something of a national sport. In a recent *The Guardian* column, restaurant critic Jay Rayner dubbed people with coeliac disease as 'attention-seeking frauds ... grown up versions of the tiresome little brats who, as children, spat out everything put their way with a shout of "I don't like it".' Comedian Jeremy Hardy recently quipped on a Radio 4 news quiz 'Bloating and wheat intolerance? When you hit your 40s, anything makes you bloated', to general laughter, but the joke wasn't exactly clear – is it really so funny to want to eat food that doesn't make you feel bad?

Often people who claim to have a food intolerance are compared unfavourably with those who are seen to have 'the real thing'. While Jay Rayner is unusually harsh in his dismissal of those with coeliac disease, journalist and columnist Rachel Cooke makes the much more common point that only those with coeliac disease can claim truly to be poorly. 'My sister has coeliac disease,' she wrote recently. 'When she first developed it, we thought she was going to die. Those who really are intolerant of certain foods tend to know about it. Everyone else is just picky or dieting by the back door.'

It is perhaps understandable that people sometimes feel irritated by those on what can seem to be faddy diets. The problem is that gluten is widespread in the modern diet, with a considerable proportion of convenient and nutritious food containing the protein. When one person decides to follow such a diet, lots of other people are affected: friends, family, dinner dates and flatmates, to name but a few.

'Dinner parties all over the country are ruined by these people,' says one general practitioner (GP). 'It's such a nuisance especially when we're out and about,' complains Sue, 32 and gluten intolerant. 'It's not just me that's affected – my partner and my friends have to make adjustments on my behalf.'

Another factor in this controversy is that opinions, often strong ones, tend to take the place of facts. That is partly because there aren't many facts available; food intolerance generally is poorly researched because clinical studies are expensive and there are few organizations that are interested in funding such research. It is widely accepted that medical training in nutrition is poor.

What's more, there are considerable corporate interests at stake – not least the bread industry, which already feels threatened by falling bakery sales.

It is against this background that this book has been written. Neither for nor against gluten, it is an attempt to provide an up-to-date assessment of the scientific evidence on gluten intolerance, much of which is not widely known. It also fills a gap in health advice today – providing guidance on how to live well and safely if you know or suspect that you have gluten intolerance.

1

Gluten free – from wilderness to mainstream in a decade

It's one of the fastest growing food choices today, and one of the most confusing. Food historians may well struggle to explain the sudden and dramatic rise in demand for gluten-free food during the first decade of the twenty-first century, as well as the astonishing increase in production.

Above all, they will seek to answer the question 'Was it all a huge scam?', as is believed by a substantial proportion of the population, including most of the medical profession? Or was there a genuine and beneficial growth in awareness of the damage that can be caused by this sticky protein in wheat and other cereals that makes up such a huge part of the modern diet.

In the early years of the decade, 'gluten free' still meant food as medicine made for people with a diagnosed illness, the autoimmune disorder coeliac disease. People with this disorder received gluten-free bread, biscuits and flour on prescription in tins from the pharmacist, and nobody was doing it for fun.

Consumers recall 'disgusting cardboard bread' that was 'just about edible if you toasted it'. Eating out was practically impossible because caterers tended to ignore requests for gluten-free dishes, regarding it as a food fad taken to extremes. Shopping, too, was a nightmare, involving a painstaking scouring of the small print on most packaged foods for any reference to gluten or the cereals that contain it.

Just a few years later, gluten free had become a supermarket favourite, housed in its own distinct shelving that was beginning to rival the size and pulling power of the organic sector. Gluten free today is a multi-billion pound industry, with more than 50 types of bread and more than a hundred brands of biscuits, cakes and pastries on sale in the UK, either through the supermarkets or online. A wide range of other gluten-free products, including pies, pastries, pizzas, soups, sauces, ready meals and sausages, are also available. It is becoming the norm for cafés and sandwich bars to offer a gluten-free option, and a handful of chefs take pride in putting at least one gourmet gluten-free dish on every menu.

So what happened? Conspiracy theorists might see the development as a wily move, masterminded by supermarkets keen to exploit the latest so-called healthy diet. One observer recalls 'something of a panic' around 2004 and 2005 as stores scrambled to fill shelves with gluten-free food – rather like the rush to go organic in the 1990s.

A great swathe of medical opinion derides this development as commercial opportunism. Leading GP, Dr Clare Gerada dismisses food intolerance as 'medically meaningless', claiming the condition is 'loved by retailers and manufacturers thanks to sales of home testing kits and free-from foods'.

Look at what happened more closely, however, and it's perhaps a little bit more complex, with a number of social and environmental changes that occurred around that time contributing to this dietary revolution.

For a start, the 'free-from' sector in supermarkets was actually initiated by a handful of staff with personal experience of gluten intolerance and the problems in finding gluten-free food. The first free-from shelves were introduced in a South London branch of Sainsbury's in 2002 by a manager who herself had coeliac disease. Tesco buyer Patricia Wheway recalls writing to her boss, Sir Terry Leahy, in early 2003 to explain that her son George was gluten intolerant and that 'it was a nightmare travelling all over the place just to find food that he could eat'. To her surprise, she was instructed to follow Sainsbury's example and set up free-from shelves for Tesco's.

Supermarket managers were finding that free-from products were proving rather popular. By 2005, market researchers were predicting a significant growth in consumer demand for free-from foods, notably gluten free, with almost every supermarket launching its own gluten-free shelves.

One of the main reasons for these confident predictions was new medical evidence showing that coeliac disease was not the rare childhood disorder that it was previously believed to be. Until scientists actually got around to measuring the incidence of coeliac disease, it was thought to affect a tiny proportion of the population – perhaps one in 2,500 people were thought to be affected.

But a major survey of all seven-year-olds in Avon, carried out by Bristol researchers and published in the *British Medical Journal* in 2004, found that this was a gross underestimate. The survey revealed that one in 100 seven-year-olds had evidence of coeliac disease. Not all of these children had active symptoms, but those who didn't had gastrointestinal markers that strongly suggested that they would develop symptoms at some time in their lives. The finding was repeated in other studies, showing that coeliac disease affects far more people than have so far been diagnosed.

The charity Coeliac UK (see Useful addresses, at the end of this book) estimates that only a fraction of coeliac sufferers are aware that they are ill. It says that around one in eight sufferers remained undiagnosed, with well over half a million Britons managing their symptoms as best they can. The success of a publicity drive to find the missing thousands was reflected in the membership of the charity (only open to sufferers with a diagnosis), which grew by an average of 900 during each month of the past few years.

At the same time, however, there is growing evidence of a quite distinct condition: non-coeliac gluten intolerance. Some experts believe that about one in 15 of the population have a problem digesting gluten. Certainly, there is now evidence that about one in ten of the population considers that they have some kind of gluten intolerance.

An even larger group of people see gluten free as a healthy choice. One in four of the population has bought a gluten-free product from a supermarket, many of whom say that their purchase is not prompted by a concern that they are gluten intolerant.

Continuing concern about sliced white bread, an undisputed hero of cheap and convenient comfort food in the 1950s and 1960s, is one of the most important influences here. Refined white flour has long been under suspicion from the growing number of followers of the 'you are what you eat' philosophy that drove the growth of the organic sector during the last two decades of the twentieth century.

'During that time, people in Britain were becoming interested in food quality, in making food choices that are made not simply on price but on the food itself: what is in it, how it is grown and how good it is for you,' says Michelle Berriedale Johnson, founder of the monthly magazine and website *Foods Matter*. 'And one of the big concerns was sliced white bread – whether eating five loaves of Mother's Pride every week was really all that good for you,' she says.

It is not just white bread that is under scrutiny. Teatime, generally, has gone out of fashion for many people. Buttered crumpets, toast and marmalade, scones slathered in jam and cream have long been seen as too naughty to be nice. The result is that bread sales have slumped by 17 per cent since the mid-1970s, with a 60 per cent drop in sales of flour over the same period.

So far, these dietary concerns fall within well understood dietary guidelines, but gluten intolerance extends further than a distaste for white bread and cakes. Wholemeal bread and pasta, the cornerstone of a nutritious diet in the view of most experts, is also under suspicion.

The media have undoubtedly played a role in raising these concerns. Women in particular increasingly see gluten as the root cause of a wide range of common symptoms that conventional medicine isn't good at treating, including bowel problems, bloating, abdominal pains, indigestion, fatigue, headache and joint pains.

This is at least partly because of increasingly wide coverage of food intolerance, generally in women's magazines and newspaper health pages. Such stories have fed into concerns about media hype, with a drive against a healthy and nutritious diet driven by celebrity endorsement – Ulrika declaring her gratitude to a wheat-free diet or Victoria pictured snacking on gluten-free chocolate biscuits.

Against that, experts argue that an increasingly well informed public is capable of making its own choices and that the move to food that is free from gluten is based on extensive if largely anecdotal information – supported by organizations and individuals who are widely gaining a reputation as authoritative and dependable, even though largely non-medical.

Foods Matter is an undisputed influence here, supporting both consumers and food manufacturers, with its monthly magazine and a website, underpinned by regular tastings of the scores of gluten-free products arriving on the market every month. These tastings led to the first *Foods Matter* Free From Awards, held in May 2008 at TV chef Anthony Worrall Thompson's shabby chic 'Notting Grill' restaurant in west London.

With pink champagne donated by Sainsbury's and assorted gluten-free goodies handed out to the assembled food journalists and a range of bakers from kitchen-table start ups delivering via the internet to the big supermarket own brands, the evening was a jolly event, run on a shoestring but with a serious message. 'The winning products are as good as and often better than the better known non-gluten-free brands,' said Worrall Thompson, handing out the awards with evident enthusiasm.

There are other influences in the field. Mario Cassar, a bio-medical scientist chemist in the National Health Service (NHS), who founded <http://www.foodreactions.org>, a website specifically targeting people with food intolerance, after a ten-year battle to cure his daughter Rebecca's food allergies with little help from the medical profession. As well as passing on his experience, the website provides a lively forum for people with allergies and intolerances to seek help themselves.

Another luminary is Professor Jonathan Brostoff, who is Professor of Allergy and Environmental Health at Kings College, London. With science and medical writer Linda Gamlin, he challenged the mainstream medical view that food intolerance was a rare condition and that most 'vague, multiple symptoms' were caused by emotional and mental problems that expressed themselves in ill health. Their book *The Complete Guide to Food Allergy and Intolerance* (see Further reading, at the end of this book) was first published in 1989 and has been frequently updated, spreading a message that for hundreds of thousands of people, identifying and eliminating the culprits of food intolerance can transform lives.

Dr John Hunter, consultant physician at Addenbrooke's Hospital, Cambridge, is the author of a series of books on the subject, most notably *Solve Your Food Intolerance: A Practical Dietary Programme to Eliminate Food Intolerance* (see Further reading, at the end of this book), as well as contributing more than 100 research papers to major medical journals including *The Lancet, Nature* and the *British Medical Journal*. He has been convinced that gluten intolerance is a far greater problem than is widely realized since he conducted an early study of 100 people with proven gluten intolerance, only three of whom had coeliac disease.

This small but influential group of experts has created a market for food without this apparently harmful ingredient that tastes good enough to eat. Alongside the *Foods Matter* Awards, it's a sign of the times that The Allergy Show, a long-established fixture in Olympia, became known as the Allergy & Gluten Free Show for the first time in June 2008. Also, the BBC Good Food Awards in October that year also held its first competition for gluten-free food.

Alongside the demand for gluten-free foods, a range of innovative suppliers has sprung up, setting about the sometimes tricky production journey to creating new gluten-free brands with imagination, commitment and a recognition that gluten-free food today must reach the highest standards.

An early enthusiast, Andrew Whitley was an artisan bread maker who had launched a successful bakery based on the premise that people increasingly believed that 'the bread on offer in the shops seemed to be making them ill'. He fell in love with Russian rye bread while he was a BBC correspondent in Moscow and returned home in 1975 to set up The Village Bakery in Melmerby, North West England, as a pioneering organic bakery.

Whitley became involved in gluten-free bread making in the early 1990s, when 'people suddenly started ringing up asking for bread made without wheat – on the face of it a tall order given that the remaining ingredients of bread are just salt and water'.

His pioneering approach was to produce 'the most nutritious food possible out of gluten-free ingredients' – rather different, he says, from the normal approach at that time when gluten-free bread was made with 'weird additives to make over-processed ingredients into superficially attractive but indifferent products'. Instead of trying to reproduce the airy lightness of gluten-containing bread, he discovered tasty alternatives, making bread with gram, chestnut or corn flour, and building on the strengths of these ingredients.

Whitley's pioneering spirit eventually led to one of the biggest commercial investments in the gluten-free market. A chance meeting with Michael Bell of Bells of Lazenby, a large craft bakery business in nearby Penrith, led to the larger company taking a stake in The Village Bakery and maintaining the products, including the gluten-free varieties, while extending commercial opportunities.

In 2005, Bells launched OK Foods, a second gluten-free brand – this time non-organic, and therefore marginally cheaper – with a £750,000 investment in a new dedicated bakery, built to clinical standards, with technical expertise and research support from Manchester Metropolitan University.

It was scary stuff, recalls Bell. His commitment, he says, was partly developed by living as a coeliac for a week: 'It made me realize that health problems don't have to be life-threatening to make life difficult.' The aim, he says, was to create products that have equivalent nutritional benefits and taste and texture as conventional foods and the results have been resoundingly successful, attracting numerous awards including the Queen's Award for Innovation alongside strong financial returns.

Roley's, another leading gluten-free brand based in the Netherlands, has won several prizes for its innovative approach to gluten-free cooking, particularly in the hard to bake area of gluten-free bread making. Its most successful bread is made from teff, a grain that until recently was only eaten in Ethiopia. It was greeted with huge enthusiasm by the Free From Food Awards – with one judge admiring its 'excellent texture and flavour' and another claiming 'If I didn't know, I would think it was normal bread.'

The rise of online shopping during this period has boosted the selling power of niche bakeries. Sue Powell was a qualified chef when she became aware of the problems that individuals with coeliac disease faced in sourcing decent, edible gluten-free foods. She decided to go into business, setting up The Gluten Free Kitchen in 2005 – 'for me, it was a personal challenge and I set about experimenting with various flours and devising a small range of recipes'.

She began production in a tiny purpose-built bakery at her home in Wensleydale, North Yorkshire in 2005, selling products like her prize-winning coffee and walnut cake and luxury bread and butter pudding through the internet. Sales went so well that she required new, larger premises in 2006, with a third expansion the following year and a doubling in the number of staff.

But there is no typical 'free-from' company. While Powell has succeeded by creating 'decent baked goods for people with coeliac disease', many other companies today are targeting a much more general market. 'We want people to buy our cakes because they like them not because they have special needs,' says Jeremy Woods, managing director of Mrs Crimble's, who decided to divert into gluten-free foods in 2005 and saw turnover in the business more than double in three years.

Which brings us up to the present – and the dilemma that so many people face in deciding whether they have an intolerance and, if so, what is causing it. That's the subject of the rest of this book.

2

Gluten intolerance – who suffers?

Ten thousand years ago, our ancestors became tillers of the land and almost certainly condemned a proportion of their number to severe bowel problems. The cultivation of cereals brought a settled lifestyle with access to highly nutritious and comforting food. But it may well have provoked a range of unpleasant digestive symptoms for a group of people who have been called 'the casualties of the slow adaptation process between the human race and wheat'.

The most extreme casualties of this intolerance, children with coeliac disease, have been recognized for more than 2000 years. The Greek physician Aretaeus of Cappadocia first described the problem in the second century AD. 'Koiliakos' meaning 'suffering in the bowels' was the name he gave to a collection of symptoms in children, of which the most significant were fatty diarrhoea, pallor, weight loss and failure to thrive.

It wasn't until much, much later, however, that the cause of this problem began to be understood. A Dutch paediatrician first made the connection between coeliac disease and the consumption of wheat during the year-long famine in the Netherlands at the end of the Second World War. Professor Willem Dicke noted that as the rest of the population suffered drastic weight loss, infant patients in a hospital ward who had coeliac disease positively bloomed. From being extremely thin and suffering severe diarrhoea on a permanent basis, they put on weight and their health improved.

His subsequent observation of their health problems returning at the end of war, when bread became available and the ward was singled out to receive the first loaves, enabled Professor Dicke to report the link between wheat and coeliac disease in a PhD thesis published in 1952.

Four years later, doctors in Birmingham, working with Professor Dicke, identified the component of wheat that caused these symptoms in children. It was gluten, a sticky compound made from two proteins, glutenin and gliadin, that together make up about 15 per cent of each grain of wheat. Imagine 'a series of tiny balloons which expand when they are inflated by the gases from fermenting yeast,' suggests Andrew Whitley, organic bread maker and author of the book *Bread Matters* (see Further reading, at the end of this book). It's this extraordinary characteristic that makes bread the wonderful food it is – 'a light, open dough structure that holds together well'.

A whole range of chewy carbohydrates from crumpets, toast and sandwiches to pizza, pasta, pies and pasties would be nothing without the chemistry that occurs when the gluten in flour is moistened and yeast is added. Other grains containing gluten are rye, barley and oats, and although they do not have the ability to form the same stretchy structure as wheat-based gluten, they are equally toxic to coeliac sufferers.

Once gluten was identified as the cause of coeliac disease, doctors set to work to find an explanation for this toxic effect. It soon became clear that this was an autoimmune disease – a type of disorder in which the body's immune system attacks its own healthy tissues. In the case of coeliac disease the tissues that come under attack are in the lining of the gut, where a healthy, normal enzyme – tissue transglutaminase (tTG) – that occupies the inside of the cells of the gut lining comes under attack as if it were a deadly microbe.

This attack flattens the villi – the thousands of waving fronds that line the gut, which boost the body's ability to absorb nutrients as the food passes through the digestive system. Once flattened, these villi are unable to absorb nutrients, including carbohydrates, fats, vitamins and minerals, causing the most serious childhood symptom: failure to thrive. And because the enzyme tTG is used to repair tissues throughout the body, the symptoms of coeliac disease can occur throughout the system, affecting bones, joints, muscles and even brain tissue.

By 1956, British doctors were able to describe in *The Lancet* the first diagnostic test to confirm coeliac disease – a simple biopsy involving the removal of a small amount of tissue from the lining of the intestine to confirm the presence of flattened villi. It was scientific evidence that proved conclusively the existence of this extreme form of gluten intolerance.

More than 50 years later, it remains the only evidence of gluten intolerance for many doctors. Yet there is now recognition that gluten is the cause of a much more common set of symptoms that are not unlike those resulting from coeliac disease, but with a totally distinct cause.

These are some of the reasons why you might suspect that you suffer from gluten intolerance.

You have coeliac disease

Until recently, coeliac disease was thought to be present from birth with symptoms showing up as soon as the child started to consume gluten-containing food. That view was disproved by a unique study carried out by scientists at Bristol University Division of Medicine and published in 2004 in the *British Medical Journal*.

A group of 5470 babies born in and around that city in 1990 have had their health meticulously studied since birth in what is known as the Avon Longitudinal Study. The findings on coeliac disease were the result of a two-stage screening of the children as they reached their seventh birthday. The screenings showed that far from being a rare childhood disease, coeliac disease affects one in 100 of the population.

The findings explained a long-recognized problem with coeliac disease – that if it was indeed a lifelong condition beginning in childhood, then why were the vast majority of people with coeliac disease diagnosed in adulthood, 'most frequently in people aged 40 to 60 years old', according to Coeliac UK (see Useful addresses, at the end of this book).

The reason is that coeliac disease needs a trigger – it may be an infection, often a simple tummy bug, or it can be stress or even pregnancy, and it must occur at a time when gluten is present in the gut. Such a trigger is harmless except in someone with coeliac-prone genes, in whom the immune system produces a reaction that has this disastrous response to gluten.

Sally
Sally suffered a severe gastrointestinal infection when she was three years old. Instead of getting better once the infection was under control, over a period of a few weeks the toddler developed the body of a starving African child with a bloated belly and stick legs. From being an energetic child, she became listless and had to be carried everywhere. Doctors were baffled, until a blood test eventually showed that she had coeliac disease – a disorder of which neither parent had heard. Once she was put on a diet that contained no gluten, Sally's health returned to normal within a week. Her younger sister Molly, then just one, was carefully monitored, and although she never suffered symptoms she too was found to have coeliac disease, also at the age of three. Two other siblings have no sign of gluten intolerance.

Margaret
Margaret was 43 and suffering from disabling swollen ankles and exhaustion when she was finally diagnosed with coeliac disease. 'I've always been pale and thin and thought that's just how I was. When I was 20, I was told to stop eating sugar and in my early thirties, I stopped eating dairy products, which I found made me feel bloated. But all the time, I think gluten was the main problem. I don't have relatives with coeliac disease. But I recently found out that there are 'hot spots' of coeliac disease around the world and the west coast of Ireland, where my mother came from, is one of them. Finding that out tied up some loose ends for me.'

So who suffers from coeliac disease?

Susceptibility to coeliac disease is inherited, although there is no predictable way in which the disease is passed down the generations. If you have a family member with the condition, then you have a one in ten chance of developing coeliac disease, with some studies suggesting that it could be even more common. Researchers have found as many as four biopsy-proven cases in a single family, although symptoms were often silent or so mild as to go unnoticed.

Coeliac disease affects all ethnic groups. It is most common in Europe and North America, but it also occurs in countries of southern Asia, the Middle East, North Africa and South America. Incidence of the disorder is also higher in people with certain health problems including diabetes, Down's syndrome, infertility, thyroid disease, rheumatoid arthritis and hepatitis.

So far, only one in eight of the more than half a million Britons with the disorder have been diagnosed. Of these, 85,000 people are members of the charity Coeliac UK, where membership is only open to people with a clinical diagnosis. A further 40,000 are thought to have been diagnosed but have chosen not to join the charity.

Of those who live with undiagnosed coeliac disease, a minority has few or no symptoms. Many others take mild to moderate symptoms in their stride as everyday upsets. Awareness of coeliac disease has increased, but it is still not high on the agenda of many doctors and is unknown in large sections of the public.

Some people may suspect they have coeliac disease but have not been diagnosed because they:

- avoid medical tests, particularly those involving a biopsy;
- have already been tested and told they are healthy; or
- have already cut out gluten-containing foods, which means

they are unable to be tested for coeliac disease because you need to be on a gluten-inclusive diet prior to testing.

You have (non-coeliac) gluten intolerance

The vast majority of people (more than 95 per cent) who go for coeliac screening test negative and are therefore frequently dismissed by doctors as having imaginary symptoms or ones that have a psychological cause. Yet there is growing evidence that non-coeliac gluten intolerance is a major health problem.

Although up to one in 100 people suffer from coeliac disease, it is now widely believed that gluten intolerance is a pyramid of suffering, with those with coeliac disease at the top and a progressively larger number of people below. Up to one in eight of the population may have a less drastic sensitivity, with a less serious long-term outcome, but one that can nevertheless cause serious discomfort.

Gluten is one of a number of types of food that is difficult to digest, and one way to measure the level of indigestibility is to determine the amount of hydrogen that is produced. Higher than average levels of hydrogen have been shown to be produced in the colon by gluten-containing foods – this is a sign that the bacteria in the colon have been exposed to food that has not been properly absorbed.

Gluten consists of many long elastic chains of proteins that can irritate the small intestine, thereby preventing the production of the particular enzymes that are needed to break down and absorb this food. As a result, the gluten tends to remain in the colon for much longer than the majority of foods do.

For most people this is not a serious problem, but there is growing evidence that gluten intolerance causes symptoms. Although these symptoms do not cause long-term harm in the way that coeliac disease does, they can be both severe and unpleasant.

Perhaps the most convincing evidence has emerged from 'blind' elimination diets that have been carried out by scientists at Cambridge University with a group of patients who claimed to have gluten intolerance. These ingenious tests allowed the scientists to monitor the impact of gluten-containing (and non-gluten-containing) food on this group without any of the participants being aware of what type of food they were consuming. The scientists were able to report that a substantial number of gluten intolerant patients were reliably developing symptoms when fed food containing gluten.

Today elimination diets remain the gold standard method of identifying non-coeliac gluten intolerance – in a situation where there is no clinical test to diagnose the disorder.

Janice, 28

Janice suffered from coeliac-like symptoms, mainly bloating and cramps followed by diarrhoea after she had a meal containing gluten. Her doctor arranged for her to have a blood test and when she went back for her results he told her to go home and make herself a nice cup of tea and a sandwich because the results were negative. She was relieved to get the all clear and was at home, delighted to be enjoying a ham salad sandwich, when the dreaded symptoms came back. She was ill for two days, missing her work.

You have a wheat allergy or intolerance

Wheat allergy is an extremely rare disorder, probably affecting a fraction of one per cent of the population. Symptoms include sneezing, itching, rashes, watery eyes, runny nose, coughing, hay fever, headaches, nausea, digestive problems, swollen limbs or general aches and pains. As with any allergy, the immune system's response to wheat is to produce antibodies as if the food were a toxic invader. Unlike a classic allergy, people who are allergic to wheat normally also have allergic reactions to four or five different foods.

Wheat intolerance is a controversial diagnosis, and there is no clear idea about what causes wheat intolerance or how many people have a genuine wheat intolerance. However, researchers recently reported in the *Annals of Allergy, Asthma and Immunology* that nearly four in every 100 of a large group of blood donors had wheat-sensitive antibodies in their blood – one marker of food intolerance.

Some experts believe that wheat intolerance occurs in people whose bodies do not produce the enzymes necessary for proper digestion of wheat. There is also a strong body of opinion that modern baking methods could be at the root of high rates of wheat intolerance.

You have a separate health problem that may involve gluten intolerance

Untreated coeliac disease may contribute to the development of a range of health problems, including osteoporosis, osteopenia and certain kinds of cancer. It is also associated with a range of disorders, including diabetes and thyroid disease. It therefore makes sense for anyone with these health problems to be tested for coeliac disease.

There is strong evidence that gluten sensitivity or wheat intolerance is a factor in IBS. There is also evidence that gluten intolerance plays a role in Crohn's disease, as well as being linked to osteoporosis, rheumatoid arthritis and thyroid disease. Some practitioners believe that fibromyalgia (a disorder involving chronic widespread pain and an excessively painful response to gentle touch) may be also partly triggered by a food intolerance. It may also play a role in depression; in a survey organized by the mental health charity MIND, as part of their Food & Mood project, nearly one in two people said that wheat adversely affected their mental state.

Other links are more controversial. There are claims that gluten or wheat intolerance plays a role in autism in genetically susceptible children, as part of what is known as the 'leaky gut' theory of the disorder. The anecdotal evidence that gluten-free diets help children with autism is sufficient for parents to feel driven to try out gluten-free diets, among other things, but it is not nearly compelling enough to convince doctors.

Indeed, a major review of the current literature, carried out by Great Ormond Street Hospital Research and published in March 2008, found that there was no evidence base to support the view that a gluten-free diet will help autistic children. But that won't convince parents, according to the National Autistic Society. 'There is an urgent need for research into the efficacy of special diets for children with autism,' a spokesman said.

Charlie and John

'No parent of a child on the autism spectrum wants to look back when the child is grown and say, "If only we had tried ...",' said Dr George Christison, Professor of Psychiatry at Loma Linda University School of Medicine in the USA and parent of a child with autism.

'It's more than upsetting; it makes me physically sick to realize that my son had been getting brain damage right under my nose with every piece of bread I had lovingly given to him,' wrote the mother of two autistic boys, Charlie and John, after she had watched a 'miraculous' transformation in her sons after she removed gluten and casein from their diet.

You reduce wheat or gluten intake as a healthy choice and find that your symptoms diminish

A national opinion poll in January 2008 reported that nearly half of sales of gluten-free food in supermarkets are to people who do not think they have any sensitivity, with only a handful of these actually believing they are intolerant to gluten. Most say that wheat and gluten products can cause them to feel bloated as well as causing abdominal pains, wind, indigestion, diarrhoea, constipation, depression, joint pain and skin irritations.

It is widely accepted that eating too much bread or pasta can produce unpleasant symptoms. A diet that is excessively high in carbohydrates encourages the body to retain fluid, for instance, which can lead to bloating; and eating poor-quality bread, which may be undercooked, can cause indigestion. There is perhaps a fine line between these normal physical reactions to an unhealthy diet and true gluten intolerance.

Julia, 56

'I cut out wheat quite regularly – it's a great way to stop myself feeling overweight and bloated. If I stop eating bread, I won't be tempted to slather butter onto a cheese and pickle sandwich or have a pizza with garlic bread on a night out.'

Lindsay, 28

'I started eating gluten-free products for three months before I got married. It was a big wedding and I was fully expecting to get as exhausted and stressed as other girlfriends who'd already done the deed. I can honestly say I had more energy in those few weeks than I've ever had before.'

3

Gluten intolerance – what are the symptoms?

'I wish I could scream this from the rooftops to help all of the others out there suffering from this miserable problem.' So says Kelly, 53, whose son George, 26, has gluten intolerance and who herself has had such desperate symptoms that she was close to having unnecessary gastric surgery.

For Kelly and George and hundreds of thousands of people with a history of undiagnosed gluten intolerance, the endless delays spent tracing the root of their 'miserable problem' can seem cruel and wasteful. On average, it takes people with this disorder an average of 13 years of seeking help before they find out what is wrong with them.

Symptoms of gluten intolerance can be confusing. Symptoms vary so widely among patients that there is no such thing as a 'typical' case of gluten intolerance. In coeliac disease, the wide variation in the type and severity of symptoms is partly explained by the extent of the intestinal damage that has occurred and the length of time for which nutrient absorption has been abnormal.

The underlying cause of identical symptoms varies dramatically. Bloating and diarrhoea may be the result of the physiological damage to the gut lining that occurs in coeliac disease. It may also be the result of non-coeliac gluten intolerance, in which no such physiological damage is present.

There is no normal age of onset and the symptoms vary throughout life. Babies and children with coeliac disease are fairly easy to identify – they are more likely to vomit and have diarrhoea, with the main symptoms being a delay in growth and failure to thrive. In adulthood, however, a whole range of problems can cause the varied signs and symptoms of poorly absorbed food, from flatulence to diarrhoea.

What's more, these symptoms are very common and have other causes, notably IBS, premenstrual syndrome (PMS) and *Candida* infection. Even more confusingly, a demonstrable link between gluten and a particular symptom doesn't necessarily mean that the link is causal – a desire for gluten-containing foods can be a symptom of some disorders such as migraine, for instance.

Louise, 39

Louise was always a pale child with mild digestive problems. 'When I started work in my twenties, I started eating junk food a lot more. I was living in a flat, eating lots of bread with sandwiches for lunch and pasta or pizza for dinner. And my favourite tipple was a pint of bitter. I started having a really upset stomach, and my energy was very low with a really wheezy tight chest. I was really pale as well; I looked like a ghost with big black bags under my eyes. I've always been very athletic and I was running a lot – I even did a couple of half marathons. But it was hard work. I would be gasping and barely able to breathe at the end. I'd go to the GP but I was always told over and over again to increase my iron intake.'

A book such as this cannot tell you for sure what's causing your symptoms, and in the first instance you should consult your doctor, rather than trying to diagnose yourself. All this book can do is provide an information base on which to plan your route to recovery. Here's a guide to tell you more about the symptoms that are frequently attributed to gluten intolerance.

Abdominal cramping

Continuous abdominal cramping with indigestion, swollen stomach and heartburn are classic symptoms of gluten intolerance.

Other causes include pregnancy, *Candida* infection, IBS and indigestion.

Anaemia

Poor absorption of nutrients as a result of gluten intolerance can cause any combination of iron, vitamin B_{12} or folic acid deficiency. Women with gluten intolerance are likely to become severely anaemic during pregnancy because their bowel is unable to absorb enough iron and vitamins to keep up with the demands of being pregnant.

Other causes include pregnancy, heavy periods, a poor or restricted diet, bleeding from the gut and (rarely) bone marrow problems.

Bloating

This is a common symptom of gluten intolerance. Poorly digested food causes a build-up of liquid or gas inside the abdomen.

Other causes include eating too much or too fast, lactose intolerance, IBS, PMS, polycystic ovary syndrome and (very rarely) a serious disease such as ovarian, liver, uterus or stomach cancer.

Constipation

This is a symptom of extreme cases of gluten intolerance.

Other causes include pregnancy, IBS and poor diet; the most frequent causes are too little fibre, PMS, old age and side effects of medication.

Diarrhoea

Diarrhoea caused by gluten intolerance results from poor absorption of fat, carbohydrate and protein, and is typically foul smelling, with greyish or pale stools that are fatty or oily and of considerable volume.

Other causes include stomach bug, *Candida* infection and IBS.

Headaches and migraine

The link between headache and migraine and gluten intolerance has been thoroughly investigated. In 2001, the journal *Neurology* reported the case of a 50-year-old man who had suffered occasional headaches for four years that suddenly worsened in frequency and severity. When he went on a gluten-free diet the headaches stopped – only to recur when the gluten-free diet was relaxed.

Another study, reported in the *American Journal of Gastroenterology* in March 2003, found that a small minority of migraine sufferers are able to eliminate or substantially reduce migraine symptoms by cutting out gluten. So far, however, a gluten-free diet is not yet seen as a first-line treatment for migraine.

According to migraine expert Dr Anne McGregor, the truth may be more complicated.

Migraine is a lengthy process with the headache part of it somewhere near the middle. The early phase frequently includes carbohydrate craving, in response to a dip in blood sugar. This is a physiological change to which people who suffer from migraine are super-sensitive. So the fact that you get migraine shortly after eating gluten-containing food doesn't necessarily mean the gluten is the trigger.

As regards other causes, a tendency to migraine is inherited, with triggers including foods such as chocolate and cheese, too much or too little sleep, hormonal imbalances, stress, irregular meals, smoking, bright or flashing lights, loud noises, intense smells and changes in weather conditions.

Infertility in women

Gluten intolerance is known to delay conception and, in severe cases, it can be a cause of recurrent miscarriage.

Other causes include ovulation disorders or problems with the fallopian tube, sexually transmitted diseases (notably *Chlamydia* infection), debilitating conditions such as cancer, low weight, obesity and fertility problems in the man.

Irritability and depression

This is a common symptom of gluten intolerance. In adults this symptom is largely caused by fatigue as a result of general malnutrition, with or without weight loss. In children, it manifests as fretfulness and emotional withdrawal or excessive dependence.

Other causes include alcohol or drug abuse, minor illness such as cold and flu, headaches or migraine, lack of sleep, PMS, thyroid disease, diabetes, Alzheimer's disease, mental health problems and learning disabilities.

Gill, 52
'If I accidentally ingest a trace of gluten, irritability is my first symptom, even before the gas and other digestive symptoms start. If I start to yell at my husband out of the blue, he nowadays asks, "What have you eaten?" It's very unpleasant because I can't really control it; I don't want to be so angry at that moment – I just am. If you have family members with this symptom, please understand that they might not be able to control the irritability at times and they might feel really bad about how they are behaving. I'm a happy and easygoing person when I haven't had any gluten accidents. And I'm obsessively careful about even traces of gluten because I hate the way I feel when I've been glutened.'

Low bone density

People with gluten intolerance are at greater risk of osteopenia and osteoporosis in the long term as a result of poor absorption of vitamin D, calcium and protein.

Other causes include low oestrogen levels after the menopause, lack of exercise, smoking and prolonged use of steroid medicine.

Low energy

The most common symptom of non-classic coeliac disease is tiredness, often due to anaemia.

Other causes include thyroid problems, chronic fatigue syndrome, PMS, sleep apnoea, narcolepsy and depression.

Mouth ulcers

Gluten intolerance is a common cause of recurrent mouth ulcers and sores.

Other causes include anxiety and stress, excessive tooth brushing, hormonal imbalance, anaemia and immune deficiency.

Muscle and joint pains

Such pains are common symptoms of gluten intolerance.

Other causes include thyroid problems, carpal tunnel syndrome, repetitive strain injury, lupus and arthritis.

Seizures

There are several reports of children and adults with seizures caused by coeliac disease, with a gluten-free diet ending seizures in those who had previously been diagnosed with epilepsy.

Other causes include epilepsy.

Skin rash

Dermatitis herpatiformis (DH) is an itchy, blistering rash that is directly linked to coeliac disease. The rash usually occurs on the elbows, knees and buttocks.

Other causes include poison ivy, hives, shingles, eczema, contact dermatitis and ringworm.

Weight loss despite a large áppetite

This is caused by poor absorption of nutrients and is often accompanied by increased fat in the stools, which can be foul smelling because they contain food that has not been absorbed properly. This is often seen as the classic symptom of gluten intolerance, yet there is now evidence that it is not the norm.

Most adults with gluten intolerance are of normal weight or even overweight at the time of diagnosis.

Other causes include anorexia nervosa, depression, medication, a serious illness, malnutrition and drug abuse.

Disorders with identical or overlapping symptoms

Irritable bowel syndrome
The UK's most common gastrointestinal disorder is suffered by nearly one in three of the population at some time in their lives. Symptoms vary from mild to severe, both persistent or during occasional flare-ups, and they include abdominal pain and discomfort, bloating, diarrhoea and constipation.

Doctors are still uncertain whether people with IBS have a physiological intolerance of certain foods or whether their gut becomes incapable of coping because of anxiety and tension. As with many people with gluten intolerance, there is no clear abnormality that shows up in tests – the function of the gut is upset but all of its parts appear normal under a microscope.

Candida *infection*
Candida is a yeast type of fungus that is normally present in a healthy person but which, when present in excess, causes itchiness, soreness and discomfort throughout the body, particularly the mouth, vagina, skin folds and groin. Other symptoms of *Candida* infection overlap with gluten intolerance and include fatigue, joint pains, irritability, digestive problems and abdominal pain.

Diseases and disorders that result from long-term gluten intolerance

- diabetes
- inflammatory bowel disorder
- lactose intolerance and other sensitivities and allergies
- osteopenia
- osteoporosis
- rheumatoid arthritis
- thyroid disease.

4

Getting a diagnosis

A gluten-free diet is not something to embark upon lightly. Before you commit to disrupting family meals, cutting out food you love and finding alternatives to an important and low-priced source of nutritious fibre, you'd do well to get a diagnosis that is as robust as it possibly can be. At the same time, however, it's worth recognizing early on that getting a diagnosis of gluten intolerance won't necessarily be straightforward.

Although far more doctors today are making it their business to learn about food intolerance, there is still considerable ignorance. Doctors frequently lack experience in and understanding of food intolerance. Nutrition is poorly covered in medical training – in the educational curriculum for both undergraduates and postgraduates. There is also relatively little hard evidence on nutritional problems in general and food intolerance in particular. Research is expensive and has to be funded, with few organizations interested in providing such funding.

As a result, some doctors still choose to ignore nutritional problems, believing they are 'overplayed' and that many readers of magazines and newspapers are made hyper-aware of normal digestive symptoms. Doctors also tend to be suspicious of disorders that cannot be precisely identified, according to Dr Shideh Pouria, a former consultant in renal medicine at Guys Hospital and now an expert in nutritional and environmental medicine. 'From the perspective of the patient, there is the simple statement that: every time I eat wheat or other grains, I get bloating or diarrhoea or migraine and I want it to stop. But clinicians have ways of characterizing these problems in terms of diagnosis depending on whether there are features of the disorder that can be shown up in the laboratory.'

Without a diagnosis of a tangible cause of the symptoms, there is a tendency for doctors to look for emotional or psychological explanations. Stressing the psychological side of symptoms can be helpful – after all, stress plays a part in food intolerance, with 'gut-wrenching' experiences disrupting the digestive system and increasing the impact of chronic digestive symptoms. Of course it can also reveal a dismissive approach to patients. Here's Dr Gerada of the Royal College of General Practitioners again revealing a somewhat patronizing view of her patients' pain. '[Food intolerance] has become part of our national obsession with finding things wrong with ourselves rather than celebrating our good health. Remember constipation, headaches and other minor complaints usually right themselves pretty quickly.'

This tendency for doctors to tell their patients worried about food intolerance to stop obsessing about their minor symptoms has been shown to be unhelpful. Research has revealed that doctors who are aware of food intolerance and have experience in diagnosing them are far less likely to consider digestive symptoms to be simply psychological. Those with experience and knowledge of food intolerance consider that up to 30 per cent of all the patients they see might attribute some or all of their symptoms to food. 'The truth is that most surveys which claim high levels of psychosomatic illness in patients who present in general practice have not taken proper account of the possibility of food intolerance,' says allergy expert Dr Jonathan Brostoff.

Louisa, 35

'I was going to see my GP for five years between the ages of 22 and 27, getting steadily more anaemic and run down. She kept giving me iron tablets when they quite obviously weren't doing me any good. I was anaemic all right and short of iron. By the time I was diagnosed, I had almost no iron in my blood. But giving me iron tablets quite clearly wasn't solving the problem.'

Raf, 32

'Three years ago, I was chatting to a friend who had recently been diagnosed with gluten intolerance and we were talking about his symptoms – and I realized they were pretty much the same as mine. I went along and had a blood test, which was positive, and the endoscopy showed I had coeliac disease. It was incredibly simple and I was completely amazed. I had never heard of coeliac disease and I didn't know anyone else who had it. In the last three years, I've discovered it is quite common in people with an Italian background, which is where my family comes from.'

So, if there is no doubt that getting properly informed about what is wrong with you is the surest route back to good health, then how do you go about getting a diagnosis? Here are the best methods currently available to pin down the cause of your symptoms.

Blood test for coeliac disease

Who should have it?

Anyone

- who has symptoms of coeliac disease;
- who has been diagnosed with IBS – one in ten people who think they have IBS actually have coeliac disease;
- who has been diagnosed with osteoporosis, infertility, type I diabetes, thyroid disease or anaemia, because coeliac disease may be a factor in all these disorders;
- who has Down's syndrome, because this group has a higher genetic risk of suffering from coeliac disease.

How does it work?

A highly reliable pinprick test kit known as the Biocard Coeliac Test Kit is available from pharmacies and supermarkets as well as online. The test breaks open the red blood cells to detect a particular type of protein – immunoglobulin A (IgA) antibodies against tTG, the presence of which is a sign of the autoimmune reaction that causes coeliac symptoms.

The procedure normally takes ten minutes to complete, at which time two coloured lines on a window on the test stick will confirm that the test has worked properly and whether the antibodies have been identified. The top line shows that the device is working; the second line shows that the test is positive, and even a faint second line counts as a positive result.

Is it reliable?

Yes – it has been validated by a series of studies. 'The gold standard for 99 per cent of coeliac patients is the presence of these antibodies,' says Tom MacDonald, Professor of Immunology at St Bartholomew's and the London University Medical Schools.

However, around one in ten people with coeliac disease are missed by blood tests, according to two major studies, one conducted in Trieste, Italy, and another involving thousands of children in Hungary who were screened at the age of six by district nurses. There are a number of reasons why you may get a false negative result (a negative result when you actually have coeliac disease).

- It is essential that the test is used at a time when gluten is still a normal part of your diet, or the IgA tTG marker will not be present in your blood. If you are on a strict gluten-free diet, then the level of IgA tTG in your blood will fall gradually and eventually result in a negative test.
- Some coeliac sufferers have a condition known as IgA deficiency, which can lead to a negative result.
- Antibody tests for coeliac disease are not accurate for children under two.
- You have non-coeliac gluten intolerance.

If you get a positive result from this blood test, you will need to see your GP, who will probably refer you for a biopsy or a capsule camera diagnosis.

Biopsy

Who should have it?

Anyone with a positive blood test.

What is it?

A thin flexible tube, known as an endoscope, is passed down your throat, through your stomach and into your small intestine. It is normally done using a local anaesthetic spray that numbs the back of the throat, or with a sedative given by injection. Small samples of gut lining are collected (biopsies) and later examined under a microscope to check for the abnormalities that are typical in coeliac disease.

Is it reliable?

Until recently a biopsy was the only way to diagnose coeliac disease, and it is still regarded as the most solid diagnostic test. It is required before you can get a diagnosis of coeliac disease, thereby ensuring that you receive the necessary long-term care and check ups as well as other benefits, including getting gluten-free food on prescription.

A biopsy will only be conclusive if the person tested is eating gluten-containing food. Once you go on a gluten-free diet, the lining of intestine can quickly return to normal and the biopsy may be negative, even though you have the disease.

Capsule camera diagnosis

Who should have it?

Anyone with a positive blood test for coeliac disease, including the small number of people who refuse to have a biopsy.

How does it work?

Called the PillCam, this 'video capsule enteroscope' is the size of a large vitamin pill and is swallowed at an outpatient appointment. Once in the small intestine, the PillCam provides high-quality images from the inside, which are transmitted to a receiver worn on the patient's belt and eventually downloaded by the doctor to a computer. The video capsule is disposable and so it does not need to be retrieved when it is passed from the body. Although approved for use by the NHS, it is still not available at every hospital.

Is it reliable?

Yes, say researchers. A comparison of the PillCam with conventional biopsy published in the *American Journal of Gastroenterology* in August 2007, found that both methods accurately detect intestinal atrophy in patients suspected of having coeliac disease.

The elimination diet

Who should do it?

Anyone who suspects that they have gluten intolerance but whose blood test or biopsy was negative for coeliac disease. Exactly how many people suffer from non-coeliac gluten intolerance is not known, but some scientists believe that up to one in seven or eight of the population may suffer from some kind of gluten or wheat intolerance. Biomedical scientist Mario Cassar says that when he was testing for coeliac disease in his laboratory at a London teaching hospital, he was concerned that only one or two per cent of the 80 or so people tested every week in his laboratory received a positive diagnosis. 'A lot of people have the symptoms but according to mainstream medicine there is nothing wrong with them,' he says.

How does it work?

It is an eating plan that involves removing specific foods or ingredients from your diet that you suspect may be causing your symptoms to see if the symptoms improve, with an extra check to see whether the symptoms recur when the food is reintroduced.

It doesn't work for everyone and can be a long process that requires a high level of commitment. It can be hard to be systematic about the foods you are eliminating and objective about the effects.

You should talk to your GP first. You can do the diet with the support of a dietician, nutritionist or allergy expert, with whom you will probably have a consultation at the beginning and end of the process.

If you decide to do it yourself, bear in mind that it can be difficult to be certain you have found the right culprit and that some people have an intolerance to more than one foodstuff.

Some pointers for those embarking on an elimination diet

- Talk to your friends or family about what you're doing.
- Read food labels carefully and work out what you can and can't eat.
- Keep a symptoms diary before you begin the diet.
- Keep a food diary to record the foods you are eating each day.
- Always consider whether your diet is balanced. A diet lacking important nutrients will cause you problems in the long term. At the beginning you'll probably feel tired and listless, so be prepared.

A true elimination diet will begin by cutting out almost all foods eaten regularly. But if you are going to test yourself, it's worth being aware that gluten and dairy products are the most common causes of food intolerance. A number of books provide a blueprint for an elimination diet including the following (see Further reading, at the end of this book):

- *The Complete Guide to Food Allergy and Intolerance* by Professor Jonathan Brostoff and Linda Gamlin
- *Solve Your Food Intolerance: A practical dietary programme to*

eliminate food intolerance by Dr John Hunter with Elizabeth Workman and Jenny Woolner.

Here is a very basic elimination diet, designed to test whether you are suffering from gluten intolerance.

Over a period of two weeks, do not have food containing gluten. Look at the labels and make sure that all the food you eat is gluten free. If after one week all the symptoms disappear, then you can be fairly sure that gluten is the problem. It may be worth having a tTG blood test if you have not already done so, although bear in mind that you must reintroduce gluten-containing foods, about five slices of bread a day for a month, before the test will work. If the symptoms do not disappear, but are reduced, then it is likely that gluten is part of the problem. If you don't experience any change in your symptoms after ten days, then gluten is probably not causing your problems.

For anyone who has successfully identified the food group that is making him or her ill, the usual reaction is to cut it out completely. However, you should be aware that one aspect of food intolerances is that you can grow out of them. Within a year, you may find yourself able to eat something safely again. But even if this is the case, it's still a good idea to limit the amount you eat.

Is it reliable?

It is probably the most reliable way to find out whether you have an intolerance to a particular food or type of food. Many dieticians warn that you may miss important nutrients by carrying out a DIY elimination diet. Clearly, it is important to be sensible and make sure that you replace important food groups, such as carbohydrates. (See Chapter 8 for information on eating a healthy gluten-free diet.)

The IgG food antibody blood test

Who should have it?

That depends whom you ask. The manufacturers and a handful of nutritionists say that anyone with suspected symptoms of food intolerance will benefit from taking the test. However, most experts say they do not work and should not be used by anyone.

Conflicting opinions on the value of IgG testing

'We all make IgG [immunoglobulin G] antibodies to food. I see no way in which this can be used to guide diet. I don't think there's any point in spending money on IgG antibody tests. The IgG antibody tests are liable to leave patients on diets that are inadequate and patients often like to think they're improving. They carry on in the teeth of very little improvement and may end up malnourished. These self-testing kits are a waste of money and should be banned.' – Dr Glenis Scadding, consultant allergist at the Royal Nose, Ear and Throat Hospital.

'We are concerned ... that the IgG food antibody test is being used to diagnose food intolerance in the absence of stringent scientific evidence ... We urge general practitioners, pharmacists and charities not to endorse the use of these products until conclusive proof of their efficacy has been established.' – House of Lords Report on Allergy, November 2007.

'The evidence for IgG antibody reactions as a basis for food intolerances continues to grow, including well designed randomized controlled trials; however, some health professionals just haven't kept up to date. Perhaps it's because a "home test" takes the power away from the professional and puts it in your hands.' – Patrick Holford, nutritionist, TV personality and author.

How does it work?

The best known IgG food antibody test, the YorkTest Laboratories FoodScan 113 (around £265), is a finger prick kit with a postal service result within ten days. The kit measures the levels in blood of IgG antibodies to 113 different types of food.

Most experts say that high levels of antibodies to a type of food can be present in the blood for many different reasons, frequently because it is consumed in large amounts or because it was introduced into your diet at an early age. It does not necessarily indicate that the body is not coping with the particular food. It may also show that the immune system is working well at clearing out any stray food proteins that have leaked into the bloodstream without being broken down.

'The claim being made in support of these tests is that people who are intolerant of a food make more IgG antibody to that food than a healthy person would. "How much more?" is a crucial question here. For a food-intolerance test based on measuring IgG levels to work, there would have to be a consistent and substantial difference between levels in people with food intolerance and levels in those who are healthy. That doesn't exist.' (An extract from Professor Jonathan Brostoff's book *The Complete Guide to Food Allergy and Intolerance* – see Further reading, at the end of this book).

Is it reliable?

Yes, according to the businesses and websites selling the tests. A single charity – Allergy UK (see Useful addresses, at the end of this book), a leading medical charity – has given the York Test its Consumer Award, which is 'given on the basis of consumer opinion, evidence of which is supplied [to the charity].'

No, according to most medical experts. They say there is no evidence to support the reliability of a diagnostic test involving IgG antibodies. Most of the 200 or so studies examining the efficacy of IgG tests are not relevant to food intolerance in adults, and early promising results in babies have now been undermined by more recent tests.

Complementary medicine tests

Who should have them?

Anyone who believes that they have a food intolerance who has trust and confidence in a complementary practitioner and who is prepared to embark on a therapeutic programme without undergoing an evidence-based diagnosis.

How do they work?

A range of diagnostic techniques is on offer from complementary and alternative medical practitioners, including acupuncture, Chinese medicine, homeopathy, naturopathy and applied kinesiology (AK).

Most complementary therapy programmes involve an initial consultation that lasts an hour and frequently focuses on favourite foods and possible intolerances. The resulting diagnoses are usually only as good as the knowledge and experience of the practitioner. In some cases, particular diagnostic techniques are used. AK is a form of diagnosis that uses muscle testing as a primary feedback mechanism to examine how a person's body is functioning. AK practitioners claim that nutritional deficiencies, allergies and other adverse reactions to foods or nutrients can be detected by having the patient chew or suck on these items or by placing them on the tongue so that the patient salivates. Some practitioners advise that the test material merely be held in the patient's hand or placed on another part of the body.

Is it reliable?

There's no evidence that any of these tests are accurate. When AK muscle testing was carried out under conditions in which both practitioner and patient were unaware of the substances being used, the responses were shown to be entirely random. Even the International College of Applied Kinesiology now states that the diagnostic method '... is not valid when used by itself.'

However, don't discount complementary diagnostic techniques. Bear in mind that you'll get an hour or so of thorough consultation with an expert who often has years of experience and extensive training behind them, and who – one hopes – has been recommended by a friend or colleague. That is something you won't get from conventional medicine. It is quite possible that an experienced and knowledgeable practitioner will be able to make useful observations and recommendations. You don't have to follow the advice blindly.

Candace, 58
'I was diagnosed with gluten intolerance while lying on my back, crooking my arm and finding that my arm muscle lost its strength when the applied kinesologist held a small jar of gluten somewhere on my body. At the time, it felt extraordinary: magical and yet completely convincing. Reading about it afterward, I began to think it was a con. And then, I recalled the consultation. This had started with me filling in a five-page checklist on food that I eat frequently and how it makes me feel. A lengthy consultation and physical examination followed before the actual test was carried out. I recall the practitioner telling me that she had decided to test for gluten when I told her how tired I became after my lunch (normally a sandwich). She also tapped my stomach and observed extensive bloating. And I have to say that coming off gluten had an immediate impact on my bowel movements. Without going on a very strict gluten-free diet, I stayed off wheat and rye products for several weeks with good results. Any time I start to feel tired or suffer chronic diarrhoea, a period of staying off gluten always helps. I was impressed by the muscle testing – but am perfectly prepared to accept this was somehow engineered and that AK as such doesn't hold water. I also believe, however, that a good AK practitioner can be very helpful indeed and that my consultation was life-changing. Perhaps it's best to regard the muscle testing as a bit of theatre, added for placebo effect. It wouldn't be the first time it had worked.'

5

What else could be causing your symptoms?

One man's meat is another man's poison, commented the historian Herodotus in 460 BC. And while many doctors still dismiss the possibility that particular foods that you eat have an impact on physical and emotional health and the method of diagnosis is controversial, Herodotus was bang up to date.

The medical profession is beginning to recognize that food intolerance is a relatively common condition, and one that is quite separate from the much more rare incidence of food allergy. What's more, food intolerance is widely accepted by complementary therapists. It's possible to consult with a member of the booming nutritional therapy industry and discover that a wide range of physical, mental, emotional and nervous system related symptoms, as well as everyday digestive problems, are signs or symptoms of food intolerance. One well known nutritional therapist lists 85 symptoms of food intolerance, including gritty feeling in the eyes, itchy red ears, difficulty losing weight, difficulty gaining weight, dizziness, dyslexia, fidgeting, irritability, lack of get up and go, and tinnitus.

Precisely for these reasons, it is worth taking a cautious, even sceptical approach to finding the cause of your symptoms. On the one hand, your GP may well be reluctant to provide support or simply too uninformed to be of much use. At the same time, therapists who frequently work in an environment where strict scientific evidence is not available may well be only too keen to attribute health problems to one or more types of foods, and the measures that they suggest can involve a great deal of time and effort.

So before considering ways of managing gluten intolerance, it's essential to consider what other reasons may be responsible for your digestive problems. Not every case of bloating and diarrhoea is a sign that you have a serious illness. It's always best to start with the simplest explanation for a problem, and the chances are that digestive symptoms like these are the result of a poor diet that for one reason or another is unbalanced or inadequate.

Bloating, for instance, is a common symptom of PMS. It can also result from constipation or from a stress-related digestive problem. It may simply be that you are eating too much, too quickly. And if food is the problem, then it may have nothing to do with intolerance as such. Too much fruit or spicy food or too many fizzy drinks can all create the abdominal gas that creates the bloat. The same is true of other symptoms that people commonly put down to food intolerance, and gluten intolerance in particular.

'Bloating and other similar digestive symptoms can be aggravated by a poor diet in general,' says Luci Daniels, a registered dietician and ex-Chairman of the British Dietetic Association. 'If you have erratic eating habits, long gaps between meals, and smoke and drink large amounts of alcohol or coffee on an empty stomach, then these problems will get worse.'

First and foremost, treat your gut with respect. It is most certainly worth making the following simple lifestyle changes before eliminating important food groups.

- Remember it's normal to feel full after lunch or dinner, especially if you've eaten a heavy meal. That can feel worse if you have irregular meal patterns where you miss breakfast and then have a large lunch, or have a larger than usual dinner. If your body is not used to the routine of digesting food, then an unexpectedly large amount will stretch your stomach muscles and cause them to expand and feel bloated. And if you allow yourself to become dehydrated or drink coffee and tea throughout the day, you are also taking risks with your digestive system.

• Consider the possibility that you are simply overloading your system with gluten-containing food. If you have toast or a croissant in the morning, sandwiches for lunch and pasta for dinner, that's an awful lot of gluten for your system to digest. It could well be that it's the quantity of gluten that is causing the problem rather than you having a genuine intolerance. According to some nutrition experts, the vast majority of people can control bloating and diarrhoea simply by eating a more balanced diet – risotto or jacket potatoes instead of pasta or sandwiches.

Commonsense steps to address digestive symptoms

For constipation
• Make sure you drink plenty of water – a glass whenever you think about it.
• Rather than cut out bread and cereals, make sure that you're eating a healthy amount of these fibre-rich foods, such as wholemeal bread and breakfast cereals, along with plenty of fruit and vegetables. 'Rather than simply adding fibre, try adding a variety of fruit, vegetable and cereal sources, ensuring a good mixture of soluble fibre (found in fruits and vegetables) and insoluble fibre (found in cereal products) – each of which has a different beneficial effect on bowel function,' says Dr Hunter.
• Try to exercise every day – it will reduce your risk of getting constipated as well as improving your mood, energy levels and general fitness.

For diarrhoea
• If you miss meals during the day and then have a large dinner, you'll over-stimulate the bowel and probably cause discomfort and diarrhoea.

- A low-fibre diet with a reduction in cereal products, fruits and vegetables is likely to help reduce chronic diarrhoea with bloating and flatulence. You can eat normal amounts of meat, fish, eggs, milk and dairy, as well as fats and oil. The low fibre diet is well described in *Solve Your Food Intolerance: A Practical Dietary Programme to Eliminate Food Intolerance* by Dr John Hunter, Elizabeth Workman and Jenny Woolner (see Further reading, at the end of this book).
- Prevent infections spreading. Ensure that you wash your hands thoroughly after using the loo to prevent you and your family from catching infectious diarrhoea. Short episodes of diarrhoea are a normal and healthy response to infection – a means of ridding the body of toxins or harmful bacteria.

For bloating
- Eat slowly. Eating very quickly and drinking fluids at the same time makes it more likely that you will swallow a lot of air, causing bloating and flatulence. The same is true if you snack or have lunch without sitting down properly and relaxing.
- Avoid fizzy drinks and sugar-free sweets containing sorbitol, mannitol and lactitol (which can produce wind and speed up intestinal movements).
- Try to keep a check on the impact of particular fruits. An increase in bloating and wind may be the result of eating too much fruit and vegetables. Cut down on pulses, dried fruits, broccoli, cauliflower, cabbage and sprouts.

Is it all in your mind?

It's sadly all too common for doctors to dismiss digestive problems as 'stress-related' or, even worse, 'all in your mind', without offering any help. The diagnosis can be right. There is a very strong connection between your mind and your gut. At stressful times, your gut may be over-stimulated and will fail to function normally.

As Professor Jonathan Brostoff points out, 'An over-active fight and flight response, perhaps as a result of long-term stress, can be responsible for chronic digestive psychosomatic symptoms including reflux, nausea and vomiting, indigestion, loss of appetite, diarrhoea and constipation.'

There is also evidence that people can become literally 'gutted' as the digestive system is overwhelmed by difficult emotions that may be impossible to express in any other way. Thus, 'gut-wrenching' experiences can cause physical changes that lead to the same kind of symptoms as experienced by those with gluten or another intolerance.

But discovering a way out of these syndromes is not easy. Getting help might involve a referral for cognitive–behavioural therapy or hypnotherapy.

It's also important to ensure that it really is all in the mind. That's not always the case, however. Professor Brostoff describes the case of Tom, who suffered debilitating migraines as a result, he believed, of the stress of working as a social worker in a hostel for alcoholics. Lacking energy and in constant pain, he moved his family to the country to escape the stress of city life and attempt a recovery. Yet it didn't happen. After a year of rural peace and quiet, Tom remained wracked by pain and with low energy, until his doctor put him on an elimination diet. 'After a week of eating nothing but meat and vegetables, he noticed a remarkable improvement: his energy restored and his head without any pain.' And the situation was reversed when Tom had a plate of pasta. 'Within an hour,' reports Brostoff, 'he was his "old self" again, and with a vengeance – exhausted, depressed, nauseated and with a throbbing pain on one side of his head.'

Deborah, 28
'I was 16 and just starting my AS levels. I'd been really down in the dumps all summer and then I got really bad gastric flu. I recovered from the flu symptoms but by then I'd developed agonizingly painful constipation, which left me stuck on the loo for hours – with completely unpredictable bouts of diarrhoea in between. There was a particularly horrible film called *Dumb and Dumber* out that summer (1994) that revolved around people not being able to get to the loo in time. Everyone else seemed to

be laughing about something that terrified me and I couldn't even tell my mother about it – I could just see my private nightmare becoming a family joke. My mother insisted I go to see the GP because I was always trying to stay off school, and she decided I was suffering from agoraphobia and referred me to a psychiatrist. I remember summoning up all my courage and telling the psychiatrist that I didn't like leaving home in case I couldn't find a loo. I didn't explain why – and he didn't ask. I think he thought it was part of my strange dysfunctional view of the world.'

Will good bacteria solve the problem?

The idea that digestive problems such as bloating and diarrhoea are caused by bad bacteria colonizing the digestive system is relatively new, resulting from studies that have built upon evidence that an eastern European diet rich in sour milk and yoghurt, replenishing the supplies of friendly bacteria in the gut on a daily basis, appears to give people longer, healthier lives.

There's no doubt whatsoever that very unfriendly bacteria such as *Salmonella* or *Campylobacter* cause severe digestive problems, notably food poisoning. Yet scientists are divided on the question of whether the absence of friendly bacteria, allowing the proliferation of marginally unfriendly bacteria, can contribute to chronic digestive problems.

A recent review of several randomized trials of the effects of probiotics on bloating by the authoritative Mayo Clinic in the USA concluded that regular intake of probiotics yielded only marginal improvements. However, another study by gastro-enterologists at Cork University College found that it was as beneficial as taking new drugs such as Alosteron, prescribed for the severe diarrhoea caused by IBS.

The problem with the theory of good/bad bacteria is that our bodies decide what is good and what is bad bacteria within the first few months of life, when the microbes that make up our own very special gut flora is established. 'Once that happens, the infant lives with the bacteria to which it has already been exposed and any other bacteria will be rejected as unfriendly,' explains Cambridge gastroenterologist Dr John Hunter. 'It's not as easy as it sounds to top up your good bacteria by introducing a new healthy strain. Our studies of patients have shown that it simply doesn't happen, at least permanently.'

That doesn't mean, he says, that having a probiotic every day won't improve your digestion. He recommends taking preparations with large numbers of living bacteria, ideally more than ten billion per gram, with the widest possible variety of bacteria present in the mixture.

'It may do and if you find that your digestive symptoms disappear with a daily dose of probiotic, then it's worth continuing. You must take it every day as the probiotic bacteria will almost certainly only exert a beneficial effect as it is passing through the gut.'

There is also good evidence to suggest that taking a probiotic during or immediately after a course of antibiotics will prevent the damaging consequences.

Could you have *Candida* infection?

Candida is a yeast that lives in the gut and in the vagina, where it normally causes no serious problems. It is part of the gut flora that colonizes the large intestine. And there is widespread concern that when the balance of this flora is disrupted, the 'good' microbes may be killed off, allowing the harmful ones – including *Candida* – to multiply, causing a range of symptoms including thrush in the vagina and digestive problems in the gut.

Writer and therapist Gill Jacobs, co-author of *Beat Candida Through Diet*, says that the microbe can proliferate as a result of an imbalance of bacteria in the gut caused by antibiotic use, steroids, stress or a diet that has too much sugar and refined carbohydrate. 'In this form, it can produce gases and waste products and sometimes alcohol. "Leaky gut" can result when it uses its roots to penetrate through the mucosal barriers and into the tissues. This allows poisonous waste products to gain access to the bloodstream, along with large food molecules that are incompletely digested,' she explained in a recent newspaper interview.

Dr Hunter, however, is less convinced. 'The symptoms of gluten intolerance are very similar to *Candida* symptoms – bloating, diarrhoea, constipation, chronic fatigue, weakness, dizziness, headaches, muscle and joint pains, breathing problems, irritability, abdominal pain and infertility – for a very good reason,' he says. Dr Hunter does not believe that yeast in the gut is the cause of the problems, nor that banning yeast as such, as the anti-*Candida* diet suggests, will help.

When a team of Cambridge gastroenterologists looked for *Candida* in the intestines of 40 patients with bloating and diarrhoea and compared them with 40 fit patients who were matched for age and sex, they found no significant difference and no signs of excessive *Candida* in either group. 'If there was an excess of yeast in the gut, then it would show up under a microscope,' says Dr Hunter.

Instead, he believes that most people with these kinds of digestive symptoms are most likely to have food intolerance. 'What happens is that the food intolerance, including gluten intolerance, causes the bacteria in the gut to ferment. It's not cutting out yeast that manages the symptoms, it's finding the food that is causing the intolerance and managing the symptoms,' he says.

Is it irritable bowel syndrome?

As many as one in five people get IBS symptoms at some time in their lives – including stomach ache, bloating, diarrhoea or constipation. It's so common that it can appear to be a 'grab-bag' diagnosis – something doctors come up with if they can't find anything specific.

Bear in mind, however, that many thousands of people suffer such intense symptoms that they are forced to consult their GP – and are taken sufficiently seriously that they are referred to a hospital gastroenterology clinic, where investigations almost always suggest that there is nothing wrong.

There is now growing evidence, however, that more than half of people with IBS are actually suffering from food intolerance as a result of a diet hypersensitivity that often develops after a bout of food poisoning or gastroenteritis. This hypersensitive reaction brings about changes in the gut bacteria that makes them respond to a 'low grade' inflammatory process that would not necessarily cause symptoms in healthy people, thereby causing abnormal fermentation in the large intestine.

Researchers at Cambridge University studied the amount of hydrogen and methane produced in the guts of people with IBS and those with no such symptoms. 'Compared to healthy people, IBS patients produced large volumes of hydrogen and little or no methane,' explains lead researcher, Dr Hunter. 'When we put them on an exclusion diet, this excess gas production fell to normal and symptoms cleared.'

Pat, 24
'I've always had a sensitive stomach, and then in May 2005 I got terrible food poisoning. I got diarrhoea every day for months afterwards – so bad that I was taken into hospital once and put on a drip. My GP said I had IBS and that it would probably go away on its own eventually and gave me an antidepressant, amitriptyline, and told me to take Imodium if the diarrhoea got too bad. I finally got myself referred to a gastroenterologist who gave me an endoscopy and a colonoscopy, and eventually one of those little cameras that you swallow. I was told that I might have "slightly" abnormal villi, which could mean I had coeliac disease or might get it in the future. I think I've probably been sensitive to gluten all my life. I've finally gone on a gluten-free diet, even though I've not been properly diagnosed as such. I'm slowly beginning to feel as though I've got more energy and less sickness.'

6

Getting treatment

Food stays in the stomach for an average six to eight hours – quite long enough for a healthy digestive system to neutralize the gliadin and glutenin, the two proteins that make up gluten, before the contents of the stomach move into the small intestine. But it's not long enough for people with gluten intolerance.

No one digests gluten quickly, but people with gluten intolerance do it more slowly. The proteins are able to persist in their undigested state for long enough for the gluten to move into the small intestine and start to cause trouble.

The classic way to prevent this from happening is to avoid the trigger. The only treatment for coeliac disease is to follow this simple rule – don't put gluten in your mouth and it won't get into your stomach.

A gluten-free diet has a dramatic impact in reversing the symptoms of gluten intolerance, often in a matter of days. Perhaps the most spectacular evidence of the benefits of a gluten-free diet has been shown in older people.

In 1994, the scientific journal *Gut* published a study showing that a group of women over 60 became significantly healthier after they were diagnosed with coeliac disease, even though the only option, going on a gluten-free diet, involved changing long-established eating habits. Far from finding this a problem, the switch to a gluten-free diet was welcomed, with the majority 'only realizing how unwell they were in retrospect, having come to accept quite marked ill health as normal.'

That finding has been repeated several times since then, showing that little recognized and long-standing consequences of gluten intolerance can be eliminated or reduced with the adoption of a gluten-free diet. Finnish researchers recently reported that five in 100 women with osteoporosis tested positive for coeliac disease, with a reduction in fractures when gluten was taken out of the diet. In 2007, Israeli researchers reported on a group of elderly people who had been diagnosed with Alzheimer's disease because of symptoms that disappeared when they were finally diagnosed and treated with a gluten-free diet.

The research shows beyond doubt that it is never too early and never too late to get a diagnosis of coeliac disease and to gain much improved health and a better prognosis for living.

For those people who have not been diagnosed with coeliac disease, however, there is another approach to gluten intolerance – neutralizing the gluten in the stomach so that it can be more easily digested and therefore prove less of a problem.

Enzyme research

An ambitious project launched at Stanford University in the late 1990s involved a unique combination of researchers from both chemical engineering and gastroenterology. And they've been hard at work ever since. The key to a potential cure for gluten intolerance, they say, is an enzyme – a naturally occurring protein that catalyses chemical reactions in the body.

Enzymes are the chemical sparks of life. Without them, many body processes could not function. Healthy digestion is dependent upon the body's secretions of sufficient enzymes, including protease, amylase, lipase, cellulase and lactase, which all break down different types of food into small components so the body can extract the nutrients it needs to build tissue and maintain health. There are an estimated 75,000 different enzymes in the human body, of which only a few dozen have been identified as these essential digestive aids.

These enzymes and the reactions that they cause can now be made artificially to top up those that the body secretes normally. Synthetic enzymes are now put to work in medicine, in synthesizing antibiotics for instance. They're also used in washing powder to break down protein or fat stains on clothes, as well as in meat tenderizers to break down proteins and make the meat easier to chew. And now it looks as though they may help with a range of digestive problems, including those caused by gluten.

In 2001, the Stanford researchers, led by chemical engineer Professor Chaitan Khosla, reported an influential study in the journal *Science*. In that report they described the structure of gluten and explained why it takes so long for people to digest it, confirming the view that gluten intolerance is a chemical engineering problem as much as it is a medical one. The approach not only provided an explanation of the problem, but it also laid the foundation for the more recent development of a possible treatment.

Khosla's group noted that two amino acids, proline and glutamine, are prevalent in gluten molecules and that the digestive tract has a tendency to lack the enzymes that can break down the bonds that they form. It showed that if the bonds linking these amino acids on the gluten protein are not present, then the digestive tract is unable to break down gluten into digestible sized chunks.

The study showed up 'the Achilles heel of gluten,' Khosla says. 'When you see that, it is relatively straightforward using one's chemical knowledge to predict how to attack it. Since then it has really been a question of what are the best weapons to attack the Achilles heel.'

A class of enzymes called prolyl endopeptidases (PEPs), a group of bacteria that seemed to be particularly good at breaking down gluten, were the first warriors to be identified. Next, in 2006, Khosla's group reported that flavobacterium meningosepticum (FM-PEP) seemed especially promising in its ability to reduce the immune system response to gluten. Another enzyme, EP-B2, a bacterium derived from barley, seemed to show great promise in cutting the gluten chain, weakening the protein to the point at which the body's natural digestive enzymes could finish it off.

Yet another study carried out at Leiden University Medical Center and published in the journal *Gut* in January 2008 identified another potential magic bullet, an enzyme known as prolyl endoprotease. Derived from *Aspergillus niger*, a rather unpleasant fungus responsible for a disease of fruit and vegetables known as black mould, it was chosen because its pH – the balance of acid and alkali – is compatible with the pH in the stomach and therefore survives the stomach's gastric juices.

'On the basis of our results, there is now a realistic chance of developing oral supplementation with an enzyme that can ensure gluten degradation in the stomach before reaching the small intestine, where it causes problems for people with coeliac disease,' says lead researcher Frits Koning.

So far, all of these enzymes have shown promise in an artificial human gut, created in a laboratory in order to track their impact on gluten intolerance, although the results have been varied. When Dutch researchers put a slice of white bread in the mix of acids in the artificial stomach with added enzyme, they found that the gluten disappeared within 90 minutes, as compared with 120 minutes when there was no added enzyme. American researchers claim that the gluten can be eliminated even faster, possibly within 10 minutes.

The next stage is a clinical trial, where the enzymes are tested in real people. It's worth bearing in mind, however, that similar enzymes are already in existence – with only anecdotal evidence that they are effective.

The best known enzyme currently available is Glutenzyme, made by the well established herbal remedy company Biocare, with the claim that it breaks down the gluten proteins found in wheat, oats, barley, rye and spelt. Another more general digestive enzyme, Spectrumzyme, also by Biocare, is aimed at breaking down gluten along with improving digestion of vegetables, fats and oils, and dairy products.

Does Glutenzyme work? Yes, according to enthusiastic contributors to the <http://www.foodreactions.org> website, which endorses the enzyme as an aid to digestion of gluten-containing food for people with gluten intolerance, at least for small amounts of gluten food or for occasions when gluten grains cannot be avoided.

Eddie

Writing on <http://www.foodreactions.org>, Eddie said, 'I have to be careful about eating gluten-containing foods like wheat, rye and barley, but I can tolerate very small amounts without any problems. If you only want to eat small quantities of gluten-containing foods such as the odd slice of bread or pastry, I thoroughly recommend the Glutenzyme tablets. I take a single Glutenzyme tablet every morning before breakfast and then have a couple of slices of brown bread (full of gluten!), without any effects for me.'

Steff

'When I first ordered the pills, I was sort of frightened to try them. I simply thought how these little white things could make a difference.

So with caution I made myself a little sandwich that I know would not give unbearable symptoms for the whole day if the pill did not work. I downed the capsule with some tea and five minutes later started nibbling my ham sandwich. Bravely I finished it and waited an hour for the bloating to kick in.

- One hour gone ... nothing – shocked!
- Two hours gone ... nothing – razz!
- Three hours gone ... nothing – very happy!
- A day went by and still ... nothing – laughing!

This was very strange but made me so happy, and surprised. This morning I had a bowl of cereal followed by jam on toast. And so far, it is a brilliant idea.'

Artificial enzymes do not seem to be effective for people with coeliac disease. Coeliac UK (see Useful addresses, at the end of this book) recognizes that the research studies currently ongoing may at some point offer the chance of less dietary restriction for people with coeliac disease, but they say that there is no such product on the horizon as yet.

'People with coeliac disease should not take enzyme supplements such as Glutenzyme, to help treat their coeliac disease,' says Coeliac UK's dietetic dietician Nicola Walpole. 'Indeed no supplements have been licensed for routine use in humans.'

Mario Cassar of the website <http://www.foodreactions.org> agrees. 'I am aware that several persons who are coeliac claim that Glutenzyme has been able to help them eat normally. But this is not recommended. If deciding so, please be careful, make sure that you do blood tests to make sure there is no damage caused by the gluten,' he says.

Julie, 35

Julie, who has coeliac disease, said 'Whenever I am glutened, I get dermatitis herpatiformis (DH) on my right hand. DH is known to be associated with coeliac disease. When my diet is perfectly gluten free, there's no DH.

I figured the only way I was going to test Glutenzyme was when eating out. There was no way I was going to deliberately eat gluten to see if it worked. As luck would have it, my sister's wedding was coming up, which meant a weekend away eating out most of the time. I took a Glutenzyme capsule before every meal.

I really, really wish Glutenzyme had worked for me. I can't imagine how freeing it would be to be able to relax more about eating out and at friends'. But sadly, on the Monday after our weekend away there was the telltale DH on my right hand. And more than a light smattering as well. Who knows, without the Glutenzyme it might have been worse, but I would recommend against coeliacs relying on this enzyme.'

Buy better bread

Yet another approach to managing gluten intolerance is to consider the quality of the gluten-containing products that are part of the problematical diet. Modern bread is a case in point.

In his influential book *Bread Matters* (see Further reading, at the end of this book), Andrew Whitley points out that gluten intolerance has only reached epidemic proportions in recent decades. 'If such a disease had existed from our earliest wheat-eating days, is it not likely that sufferers, not knowing the cause or not having enough other food to eat, would have fared rather badly in the evolutionary stakes?' he asks.

A more plausible explanation might be that widespread gluten intolerance today could be the result of 'a combination of changes in wheat itself and a move to fast fermentation using commercial yeast that has rendered the bread indigestible to certain individuals who may, granted, have had some genetic predisposition against gluten.'

He points to recent research showing that lactic acid bacteria may be capable of deactivating the very substances that cause gluten intolerance. In 2002, Italian scientists used sourdough lactic acid bacteria to neutralize some wheat gliadin. And in 2004, Japanese scientists reported that lactic fermentation of soy sauce removes allergens from wheat, at least in laboratory conditions. More remarkably, he says that people with gluten intolerance have been shown to have no reaction to Italian bread made with dough that has been fermented with selected sourdough lactobacilli.

This experiment, says Whitley, is 'a ray of hope' for people with gluten intolerance. 'It suggests that everyone should be able to eat wheat and rye bread if we get the bread making right.'

Managing vitamin deficiencies

Many of the symptoms of gluten intolerance could also be caused by nutritional deficiencies. These can affect people even after they start a gluten-free diet and include the following symptoms:

- depression and brain fog, which are symptoms of B vitamin deficiency;
- lack of stamina and feeling overwhelmed, which are caused by iron deficiency;
- muscle cramping, twitching, muscle pain, high blood pressure and heartburn, which can be caused by magnesium deficiency; and
- osteoporosis, which can result from calcium and vitamin D deficiency.

It is possible to consult a nutritional therapist and to be screened for these kinds of nutritional deficiencies, with a strong chance that it will be recommended that you start taking a wide range of vitamin and mineral supplements in order to achieve an optimal diet.

There is now considerable evidence, however, that vitamin supplements are not effective in improving health. Mineral supplements are different. It is often a good idea to take supplements to balance intake of iron, folate, magnesium and calcium.

However, the best way to overcome mineral and vitamin deficiencies is to eat a healthy balanced diet. Ask your GP about whether it is worth seeking a referral to a dietician who can advise on achieving a healthy balanced diet.

Acupuncture

In Chinese medicine, gluten intolerance is seen as one of many health problems caused by *Qi* or energy deficiency in the spleen system. The health of this energy system is thought to determine the body's ability to absorb nutrients, because a healthy digestion is reliant on the spleen's ability to transform and transport food and fluids.

With gluten intolerance, the spleen system becomes or is already compromised, depleted and deficient in many ways.

An additional condition known as 'dampness' can be involved, which slows down the flow of *Qi* even more.

Acupuncture can work to help strengthen and build the *Qi*, unblock and move stagnant *Qi*, resolve dampness and restore balance in the entire system.

A good acupuncturist will use specific acupuncture points to nourish and tone the spleen system, smooth the liver system and heal damaged tissues. As well as alleviating pain and other symptoms, this should work in the long term to drain dampness and help to normalize stomach acid secretions.

Always make sure that anyone you consult for acupuncture is properly trained and has experience of treating gluten intolerance.

7

Is gluten good for your health?

When novelist Kingsley Amis invented the Boozing Man's Diet in his book *Everyday Drinking*, first published in 1983, he could not have predicted how popular his regimen would become. His plan for staying slim without reducing alcohol intake was devastatingly simple – cut out bread and order food you don't like in restaurants.

If the second measure has not really caught on, the idea of cutting out bread to stay thin – or at least healthy – has proved a hit. The likes of Ginger Spice and Ulrika Jonsson have made a gluten-free or bread-free diet their number one health tip; wheat-based products stand condemned as stodgy and fattening, while wheat free brings vitality and glowing energy. Gluten is also on the 'to bin' list in the regular detox diets followed by actress Gwyneth Paltrow, who cuts out 'grains with gluten' alongside most other foods in the detox menu that allows her 'salad with carrot and ginger dressing' for a week twice a year. She may look well on it, but is this preference a healthy choice or the trigger for a dangerous celebrity-led, media-driven health fad?

According to a significant and vocal body of opinion, it's the latter. Bread, after all, is the staff of life. The Egyptians paid it as wages. For the Romans it was a form of dole, and the French revolution was a response to its disappearance from the shops. It was the world's first 'convenience food', able to be produced on a large enough scale to feed an industrial workforce. And for many well known nutritional experts, bread remains an essential element of a healthy diet. For a start, white flour has been compulsorily fortified with calcium, iron, thiamine and nicotinic acid in the UK since the Second World War.

At the same time, bread contains high levels of complex carbohydrates, which keep energy levels high and can help maintain a healthy weight. With evidence that the only proven strategy for long-term weight loss is a balanced diet that is low in fat and high in carbohydrate, it can be claimed that bread – along with other carbohydrate-rich, wheat-based convenience foods – is one of the easiest and the cheapest ways to maintain a healthy weight. The problem with such claims, however, is that as well as being a significant part of the Western diet, bread and other bakery products are also at the centre of a massive commercial industry. And with little independently funded research into this key area of nutrition, it can be difficult to disentangle commercial messages from truly independent health education.

Certainly, bread, especially the wholegrain variety, is a great source of fibre, preventing constipation and keeping the digestive system and bowels healthy and thereby preventing chronic diseases such as coronary heart disease, diabetes and colorectal cancer.

It is this wealth of health benefits in what must be the ultimate convenience food that makes nutrition experts so concerned about 'uninformed' health choices to give up wheat.

'Teenagers especially can end up getting in a real mess with their diet if they think they have an allergy to wheat,' warns nutritionist Jane Clarke, writing in a national newspaper. 'They can end up going the whole day just having drinks and crisps and anything sweet they can grab in the belief that they are opting for a healthy life-style.'

'Cutting out wheat is almost always an extremely bad idea – at best it will lead to mental and physical underperformance but at its worst this type of fashionable fad will set women on the slippery slope toward an eating disorder,' says Professor Tom Sanders of the Department of Nutrition & Dietetics at King's College London.

As is often the case, much of the research underpinning these concerns – or at least the promotion of research findings – is corporate. Professor Sanders' warnings are widely quoted in a Grain Information Service report published in 2008, entitled *Food Allergy or Fashion Victim*. It is a series of studies, carried out by the Flour Advisory Bureau (FAB) over several years, that has attracted attention to fears about the consequences of cutting bread out of the diet without proper planning. As its name implies, FAB is funded entirely by the bread industry, and inevitably the inclination is to wonder: Well they would say that, wouldn't they? One survey shows that four out of ten women eliminate specific foods from their diet, with half of them doing so without planning on how to replace the nutrients they are losing or taking dietary advice about making such whole-scale changes to their diet.

While women in a 2008 survey 'are now far more knowledgeable about their own health than in previous years', they still continue to demonstrate 'considerable confusion and misinformation regarding nutrition and diet'. Nine out of ten women had no idea of the difference between a food allergy and an intolerance, for instance.

Another FAB survey of GPs' attitudes was equally worrying. Nine out of ten family doctors express anxiety about 'fashionable' diets that encourage their patients to eliminate foods such as wheat without a medical consultation, thereby putting their health at risk by depriving themselves of important nutrients. Over a third of GPs questioned were particularly worried about 'questionable' and 'potentially harmful' advice given to women by poorly qualified nutritionists and health practitioners, frequently via the media.

Many women run into dietary problems by eliminating wheat and gluten products without proper advice, according to the British Nutrition Foundation, an entirely independent scientific body that is, nevertheless, at least partly funded by the food industry. 'Elimination diets are supposed to be a short-term exercise rather than a permanent solution,' explains Dr Judy Buttriss, the British Nutrition Foundation's director of science. 'They should only be used by health professionals with the specific intention of isolating a problematic food through a process of carefully reintroducing foods over no more than two weeks.'

She continues, 'But this very controlled diagnostic process has been misapplied by unqualified individuals who now preach elimination diets as a long-term dietary solution for everything from weight-loss to intolerance. Women should be extremely cautious of any diets like these and especially wary where they are given no advice on how to replace the nutrients they will be losing with alternative foods.'

Katy, 22

Katy worried that she was getting 'stomach noises' after eating anything containing gluten. 'It wasn't serious. There was no stomach pain, no constipation, just extremely embarrassing noises and slight discomfort.' She had already cut out dairy products because of digestive problems. Now she cut out gluten and found that things improved for a while, until the noises started again. I was ready to pull my hair out and felt unable to go on dates until it was resolved. I kept a food diary, and finally went to my GP for a definitive coeliac test against gluten. It came back negative, nor did I have any parasites which can also be a cause of digestive problems.'

Her GP referred her to a dietician, and with the help of the food diary she was able to make progress. 'My fibre intake was very low – mainly because I had cut out wheat products, which are naturally high in fibre. So after the "OK" from the gluten test, I decided to reintroduce wheat into my diet and increase my fibre.'

'I began with half a slice of bread and increased it a little at a time. I'm also eating more fruit and vegetables and taking exercise. After just two days I felt totally different – less tired, more energized and the stomach noises had almost totally gone. I then got brave and reintroduced cheese/yoghurt, and I still feel great. And I feel a lot better and the noises have stopped too.'

Market research commissioned by the gluten-free food industry seems to back up these concerns, at least in the sense that an increasing number of people are making decisions about their diet without recourse to health practitioners. The rapidly expanding gluten-free sector is not driven by people with a medically recognized problem, whether coeliac disease or gluten intolerance.

Seven out of ten customers simply want to eat less wheat and gluten, seeing gluten-free food as a healthy choice but not one that they have no option but to eat. In other words, most people buying gluten-free foods are exactly the people causing such concern to diet experts. According to market researcher Angela Mumby of Food Ambitions, this group is young (under 45) and far more likely to rely on self-diagnosis or the internet rather than their GP or government websites or pamphlets as a source of information on dietary matters.

'We seem to live in an increasingly less certain and trusting world in relation to food,' she comments in a report widely quoted within the industry. 'People are making their own minds up when it comes to diet and lifestyles and using an eclectic mix of information sources to choose how they live their lives and what products to consume. Whether their new sources of information are more reliable is another matter but consumers do want to find their own way on diet and nutrition rather than be told what they should do.'

So what is happening here? Are large numbers of people really behaving irresponsibly and putting their health at risk on the basis of inaccurate information 'spun' by celebrity reports? Or are mainstream nutritional experts themselves ignoring data that raise doubts about gluten in the modern diet?

One controversial item in the world of dietary advice is the white sliced loaf. Widely mocked by 'foodies' as tasting like cardboard without cardboard's nutritional benefit, white sliced bread avoids being panned by dietary experts, largely because white flour is compulsorily fortified in the UK.

Yet while it is technically correct that white flour is fortified, critics of the modern baking industry say the claim should be put into context. In his book *Bread Matters* (see Further reading, at the end of this book), Andrew Whitley, founder of the celebrated organic Village Bakery in Melmerby, points out that roller-milling wheat into white flour removes 60 per cent of the naturally occurring calcium in the grain. 'In 1941, the Government forced a very reluctant milling and baking industry to accept mandatory fortification with chalk,' he says. 'It is chutzpah of a high order for the Flour Advisory Bureau now to claim that white bread is a good source of calcium without so much as a murmur either of its former opposition to fortification, or of the possibility that added chalk may not have the nutritional integrity of the naturally occurring calcium.'

What's more, says Whitley, there are other nutrients in wheat that are lost in roller-milling that are not made good in fortification. 'It is at best opportunistic and at worst deceitful for the industrial milling and baking industries to make nutritional claims about UK white flour being a "good source" of any nutrients purely on the basis of mandatory fortification.'

Alongside fortification, the baking industry, frequently with the support of nutritional experts, makes much of the fact that bread is cheap. The lead story in the summer 2008 issue of *Update*, FAB's publication for journalists, is headlined *Bread: Value for Money*. The article, written by Fiona Hunter, FAB's consultant nutritionist, points out that white bread in particular is a cost-effective way to consume minimum levels of vital nutrients, which is especially important in a recession. 'In an era when every penny spent in the grocery shop is put under the microscope, it's worth reminding customers that bread represents excellent value for money,' she says.

Yet at a time when the rationale of 'the cheaper the better' is under scrutiny in so many other areas of our food shopping –

notably chicken and pork – it's worth considering whether the FAB claim really holds water.

Andrew Whitley, one of the few 'real bread' experts to have provided a detailed critique of what he calls 'the madness behind the adulteration of our most basic food', argues that it is the very determination of manufacturers to create the cheapest possible product that has caused bread sales to fall continuously over the past few decades.

Even 'healthy-eating brands adorned with images of nature and vitality that make detailed claims about the virtues of this or that added nutrient,' he says, are 'barely distinguishable from others being sold at less than the price of a postage stamp.'

Bread consumption, he claims, has slumped because 80 per cent of bread sold in the UK has 'the pappy texture and bland flavour of the Chorleywood Bread-making Process – a method using lower protein wheat, a substantial assortment of additives and high speed mixing, creating bread that stays fresh "day after depressing day". Most of the rest, including the so-called healthy eating brands, use activated dough development that also relies on large numbers of additives.'

Both methods, he says, produce bread of 'phenomenal volume and lightness with great labour efficiency and at low apparent cost.' Yet there is growing evidence, he says, 'that it has also rendered bread indigestible to certain individuals who may already have some genetic predisposition against gluten.'

Whitley argues that it is modern bread rather than our genetic intolerance of grain that is the problem. He points out that gluten intolerance has been a significant problem for around 50 years. 'If such a disease had existed from our earliest wheat-eating days, is it not likely that sufferers, not knowing the cause or not having enough other food to eat, would have fared rather badly in the evolutionary stakes?'

The fact that gluten intolerance is increasingly common, he says, shows that a good many of the genes have survived. Most worrying, he says, is that recent research indicates that one enzyme quite widely used in the food industry – transglutaminase – can generate in the human gut the epitope of gliadin that is toxic to people with coeliac disease and other intolerances.

Whitley wants to see minimum nutritional standards for bread-making wheat, with millers using flours that conserve more of the nutrients naturally present in the grain. Industrial bakers should also come clean about the additives that go into their bread.

Most of all, he says, 'we urgently need research to compare the digestibility and nutrient availability of fast-made and long-fermented breads. If it turns out that putting the time back into baking (and removing the additives) could make bread good again – even, perhaps, for coeliacs – not only would public health improve, but we might learn that the less we try to manipulate food the more likely it is to nourish us.'

So would gluten intolerance disappear in a world in which Chorleywood's additives, enzymes and high-speed dough are replaced by bread made by artisan bakers or baked at home? Will our digestive systems improve if the dough is left to ferment over periods long enough to make available as many nutrients as possible?

Some scientists claim that there is evidence that grain itself is unhealthy. According to proponents of the Stone Age or Paleolithic diet, the only healthy choice is to stick to food that can be either hunted or gathered – meat, fish, fresh fruit, vegetables, nuts and eggs. The rest, particularly grains, is not suited to our genetic make up. And it's certainly not an essential part of our diet.

Developed in the 1990s by a group of American clinical nutritionists, the fundamental principle of the Stone Age diet is that many chronic diseases of Western civilization have been caused by 'an evolutionary collision between our ancient genome (genetic make-up) and the nutritional qualities of recently introduced foods.'

The phrase 'recently introduced' requires explanation. The Stone Age diet is not targeting foods introduced during the past decade, or even the past millennium. Rather, the principal underpinning the diet asserts that the introduction of agrarian farming, bringing plentiful grain-based foods into the diet 10,000 years ago, happened too recently on an evolutionary timescale for the human genome to adjust. Since the introduction of grains, according to Stone Age dieticians, the human race has decreased in height and become more vulnerable to infectious diseases as well as arthritis, hypertension, heart disease, stroke, depression, schizophrenia, cancer, osteoporosis, rickets and anaemia.

Because most of our evolution took place without wheat, they say, it cannot really be essential for us to eat it. A substantial number of people in the world rarely if ever eat wheat. In Kenya and Zimbabwe the staple food is maize, often eaten with beans, or eaten as polenta or porridge. While Italy's biggest export is wheat-based pasta, the staple in many parts of the country is also polenta made from maize.

Uganda's staple is cooked green bananas, often eaten with groundnut sauce. In the Caribbean, plantains are an easily prepared source of starch. In India, rice with lentils is the most common carbohydrate, while in northern Canada fish is the staple food, and teff in Ethiopia.

Dr Ben Balzer, an American doctor and leading proponent of the Stone Age diet, says that grains are anti-nutrients that are packed full of toxic proteins to discourage predators – some of which persist at low levels when the grain is cooked. We don't eat apple seeds, he points out – we enjoy the fruit and excrete the seeds, bringing the possibility of a new apple tree. The seed in grain has exactly the same purpose – it is intended to perpetuate the lifecycle of the plant, but it's also close to the ground and therefore easy to eat and in a vulnerable position.

'Therefore,' he continues, 'it has been loaded with toxic proteins to discourage predators. Grains are full of enzyme blockers that are effectively poisons and lectins, natural proteins that break down the surface of the small intestine, stripping it of mucus and causing the cells to become irregular and leaky. You may be surprised to learn that uncooked flour is very toxic – please don't try eating it as you become very sick. And yes, I don't recommend *al dente* pasta.'

Grain-based foods also have a high glycaemic index. In other words they cause sugar or energy spikes, which create a vulnerability to infection and disease. They are also low in vitamins, minerals, antioxidants and phytosterols – they are 'the original empty calories', Dr Balzer says.

Once you start looking at bread as the enemy, you don't have to search for long to find claims that wheat-based foods are pretty well nutrient-empty, potentially indigestible and slightly toxic even when baked, at least for a minority of people.

'I would always refuse to eat wheat,' says Barry Groves, author of *Trick and Treat: How healthy eating is making us ill* (see Further reading, at the end of this book), a book that received widespread, if sometimes sceptical, publicity when it was published in 2008. 'Wheat collects bacteria and dirt as it grows and it's impossible to clean,' says Groves. 'Then stored in silos, it's a haven for mice and rats so it gets sprayed with insecticides. Put wheat flour under the microscope and you'll see traces of rat faeces.'

But if we are not convinced by the claim that our morning toast has traces of rat faeces, Groves has accumulated a potentially worrying collection of research papers that call into question claims that gluten-containing food is healthy.

One group of researchers have attempted to investigate the nutritional value of wheat- and gluten-containing products by comparing the health status of people who have coeliac disease and are therefore on a gluten-free (and wheat-free) diet with the 'healthy' population that consumes gluten regularly. The following studies, all published in peer-reviewed journals, show that people who avoid wheat and other gluten-containing foods appear to be considerably healthier in a number of key areas than general population norms.

Thus, one major study found that the risk of two killer diseases, breast and lung cancer, fell dramatically in people who avoid gluten. Nottingham epidemiologist Professor Joe West, reporting in the *British Medical Journal* in September 2004, compared the health profiles of nearly 5,000 people with coeliac disease with 23,620 'matched controls' over a period of two years. During the first year after diagnosis and therefore going on a gluten-free diet, people with coeliac disease had a slightly increased risk of a range of diseases compared with the healthy controls. After that point, however, there was a sudden decline in the incidence of cancers in the gluten-free population, with individuals in this group having a third of the risk of developing the cancers compared with the healthy population.

The dramatic reduction in lung cancer cases might be explained by the fact that people with coeliac disease were less likely to smoke, he says. However, the reduction in breast cancer cannot easily be dismissed. 'The findings are of interest, because there are clearly factors at work that seem to protect people with coeliac disease against breast cancer.' Of three factors – genetic and environmental as well as nutritional – he says that the gluten-free diet most clearly differentiates the people with coeliac disease from the general population.

Barry Groves believes that people with coeliac disease might get this extra protection by cutting out the junk that is contained in many gluten-containing convenience foods, which they are forbidden alongside bread and pasta. 'When people are diagnosed with coeliac disease, they cut down on bread, pasta and packaged foods with hidden gluten such as modified starch. As a result, their blood glucose levels fall and as high levels of glucose increase the risk of cancers, merely the change of diet following diagnosis would reduce their cancer risk,' he says.

Another study suggests that adults on a gluten-free diet are also less likely to have high blood pressure compared with the general population. Yet another series suggests that gluten may trigger or worsen rheumatoid arthritis, with 'numerous case studies reporting alleviation of arthritis symptoms with grain-free diets', according to Groves. There is even evidence of a 'gluten-sensitive subset of people with schizophrenia', who appear to process gluten in a way that exposes their brains to certain very psychoactive substances that are now known to exist in these foods.

And the research is continuing. In the most recent paper, published in March 2008, rheumatologists at the Karolinska University Hospital in Stockholm reported that arthritis sufferers who went on a gluten-free diet had 'significantly lower cholesterol and body weight – and therefore a reduced risk of heart disease.' A gluten-free diet could be used to improve the long-term health of people with rheumatoid arthritis, say the researchers, in a paper published in the journal *Arthritis Research & Therapy*.

None of this research is in any way conclusive, but it does suggest that Kingsley Amis may have been on to something. It could be that however cheap, convenient and apparently nutritious it is, for some people gluten is not a friendly food, at least not in the quantity that is currently consumed.

8

Eating gluten free

'Go on, try the gluten-free baguette! – that was the ominous dare that crept around the tasting table.' So begins a review in the monthly journal *The British Baker* of gluten-free foods or, as they describe it, 'that unique niche: bakery products for people who cannot eat bakery products'.

Perhaps not surprisingly, the British bakers were not impressed by the baguette. 'On the surface, this curio seemed inviting enough: a dark crust, a slash down the centre, your standard bake-off quality baguette. But on the inside lurked something more akin to petrified loft insulation, with the mouth-feel of running your tongue up a brick wall,' was how they summed it up.

For anyone with a taste for a French baguette or bread of any type or nationality, cutting out gluten is tough. It is hard to find one ingredient that replaces gluten's function in baking and still get bread, cakes or biscuits that taste anything like the real thing. Poor gluten-free products taste gritty, dry and heavy. Alongside bread, biscuits, cakes, pasta, pizza and beer (made from wheat), most convenience and processed foods are off the menu. Anything with additives or added seasonings should be seen as suspect. And some of your favourite foods are almost certain to be off limits: fruit gums, liquorice, dry roasted nuts and Worcestershire sauce, to name just a few.

You'll have to face up to the fact that many restaurants are out of bounds – both for you and anyone who wants to eat with you. So are the majority of cafés, unless you're just there for a hot drink that's not from a vending machine. You can't even consider normal sandwiches or crisps or pizzas – the kind of food that you can eat on the hoof and that so often eases life while you're working or travelling.

Yet you can be positive about going gluten free – you can choose to focus on what you can eat rather than what you can't, to consider this as an opportunity to eat a healthy, perhaps even healthier diet. There's even a view that you could become a 'better' person by eating gluten free.

Julie Meyer, American acupuncturist and 'a gluten free mom raising a gluten free child', says that abstaining from 'sticky', 'full-making' gluten could have spiritual side effects. The current near-epidemic of gluten intolerance, she suggests, is 'warning us of a major weakness in our micro-cosmic system – the body. We're too full. We need more space, more emptiness, less puffed-up-ness in our lives. Abstaining from gluten – that which fills, expands, makes sticky and full – is resonant with the deepest origins of being and with current nutritional wisdom.'

Back on planet earth, the good news is that the problems of eating gluten free have been addressed by a wide range of experts. First and foremost among them are those who live with gluten intolerance and who have devoted a considerable amount of time to tracking down alternatives to favourite foods: gluten-free beer that can be delivered, varieties of Walkers crisps that are gluten free (prawn cocktail and plain), cakes that get the approval of the families of people with gluten intolerance as well as dieticians and nutritionists.

For the first time in 2008, gluten-free food was featured at the BBC Good Food Show in Olympia. Gluten-free pickles, pastas, pestos, spices and sauces, as well as breads, pizzas, flours, gnocchi, sausages, chocolates, cakes, biscuits, breakfast cereals and liqueurs were among the foods on show.

Here's a meal-by-meal summary of how the experts say you can make life easy.

Julie
'I always say that I actually like being gluten intolerant because it steers me away from the processed junk that is everywhere in our toxic culture. When I think about it, I only ever crave gluten-free bread or muffin equivalents when I'm caught up in the manufactured sense of urgency of that culture – what you might call the sticky puffiness of our modern lives.'

Louise, 39
'It was very hard giving up wheat – especially on holidays. I love to get away for the weekend, walking during the day and sampling the local beers in the evening. But you can't just wolf something down or grab a sandwich on the run. You can't even have a salad in case there's gluten in the dressing. And that's a nuisance, especially when I'm out with my partner or friends. They suffer too.'

Staying healthy eating gluten free

By embarking upon a gluten-free diet, you're eliminating one of the best sources of starch (a vital source of energy), as well as protein, vitamins and fibre. Here are the best alternatives to these essential elements of our diet.

Starch
Try alternative grains such as maize, millet, rice and quinoa – all more nutritious than the more obvious alternatives such as refined rice, corn and potatoes. Other starch-rich foods include lentils, beans, sweet potatoes, parsnips, plantains, green bananas and yams.

Protein
Nuts, seeds, eggs, meat, fish and pulses provide plenty of protein.

Vitamins
Wheat flour is naturally rich in B vitamins and vitamin E, and is fortified with calcium, iron, and the B vitamins niacin and thiamine. Most gluten-free flours are not. What alternative sources of these essential nutrients are there?

- calcium: dairy, sardines, watercress, figs, almonds and nuts
- iron: red meat, liver, kidneys and sardines
- B vitamins: black-eyed beans, brown rice and Marmite
- vitamin E: nuts and avocados.

> *Fibre*
> If you substitute gluten-free alternatives for wheat-based bread and pasta, you may be at risk of eating too little fibre. Rice, potato and tapioca flour, commonly used in commercial gluten-free products, are all low in fibre. Get extra fibre by eating plenty of nuts, seeds, vegetables and fruit, as well as gluten-free wholegrain such as brown rice, buckwheat and millet. This is particularly important for older people, who are at greater risk of constipation.

Breakfast

For anyone who likes toast with their coffee, going gluten free is likely to be challenging. Breakfast is commonly gluten rich in the modern diet, unless you're going to stick with naturally gluten-free cornflakes or more old-fashioned alternatives such as bacon and eggs, with devilled kidneys on the side.

When Peter Thomson was diagnosed with gluten intolerance, he wrote his own cook book *Gluten-Free Cookery* (Hodder Arnold, 1995), while his website (<http://www.peter-thomson. co.uk/glutenfree.index.html>) – featuring recipes and an online support group – has become one of the best established and most respected gluten-free resources.

For breakfast Peter favours kedgeree with rice and ham or teff porridge made from the versatile, healthy grain that until recently has only been available in Ethiopia but is now widely available on the internet (<http://www.innovative-solutions. org.uk>). His favourite is a kind of muesli based on easycook brown rice with olive oil and raisins, with jam and a spoonful of yoghurt. 'The jam is homemade with fruit from the garden because I don't like all the additives and poor flavour from bought jam. And yes, it keeps me fit and walking over the moors every weekend.'

Lunch

This is potentially one of the most problematical meals, especially if you are at work or travelling. Part of the problem is that lunch for many people means a sandwich, a tasty, convenient, nutritious and filling snack. So what's the alternative?

What's the alternative?

The gluten-free bread available in supermarkets can be disappointing: too heavy, too crumbly and too dry. Most have to be 'refreshed' in the microwave before consumption, which is a drawback for people who want to eat the bread at school or at work.

Bread mixes rather than ready-made bread seem to be the preferred solution. The overall winner at the prestigious 2008 Foods Matter Awards was Roley's teff flour mix (<http://www. roleys.com>) – a bread mix based on maize and teff, a highly nutritious seed grown in the mountains of Ethiopia.

And Roley's mix doesn't seem to be a one off. Other bread mixes also attract glowing references. Mixwell of Sweden (<http://www.mixwell.se>) is another award-winning producer, with a large range of gluten-free bread mixes and flours. Sheona Viandello of Drossa Ltd, who imports the brand to the UK, says she prefers to make the mixes up by hand as it means she can adapt them. 'For example I add dried fruit and nuts to the Spicy Bread mix and bake it in foil pudding basins (makes a great fruited loaf); add herbs to white bread for a tasty alternative; the seed bread is great on its own (and it keeps for several days) but I sometimes also add some raisins to the mix; and use pizza mix to make delicious Focaccia type bread with added dried tomatoes or olives,' she explains.

There are now bread makers on the market that have gluten-free settings – for instance the latest Panasonic bread maker (<http://www.panasonic.co.uk>). Remember to buy a spare pan and paddle to be used only for gluten-free bread if you're also planning to make bread from wheat flour.

Penny

Penny, writing on the internet: 'My husband is coeliac and for a few years he put up with the prescription bread – Juvela and Glutafin. However, after trying the Glutafin Fibre Bread Mix (<http://www.glutafin.co.uk>), I have had amazing results. It's simple. You just follow the instructions on the pack, chuck it in and set on "rapid bake". One hour and 55 minutes later, you have a beautiful, tasty, normal looking loaf that you can cut nice big slices from. It's best made a day before use but the smell is often too tempting to wait a day!'

But you don't have to eat gluten-free bread. An alternative, tried and tested solution, which works for gluten-eating people as well, is to make a packed lunch out of leftovers: leftover chicken and roast potato with slices of cucumber and tomato; tinned salmon, with leftover new potatoes, Chinese leaves and a stick of celery; or kedgeree with diced egg and cheddar cheese. Or you could put nuts and seeds in instead, or have a handful of nuts with some fruit.

At home there is a huge range of alternatives to choose from. Kate Chan, an American who was diagnosed with gluten intolerance in October 2000 three weeks before her wedding, now writes an inspirational blog (<http://www.glutenfree.wordpress.com>). After several years of extreme illnesses, exhaustion, lack of energy, inability to focus and unexplained tummy issues, she writes about her determination 'to bake, cook and enjoy life again'.

Being gluten-free and planning lunch as a student and starting work has forced her to become more organized and thorough about her plans for the day. 'I no longer just "wing it", but make sure that I have a plan for myself so I don't feel deprived or annoyed ... or downright crabby at work.'

Here's an abbreviated list of her favourite lunches.

- green leafy salads
- quinoa salads or quinoa tabbouleh
- fruit: grapes, cherries, oranges, blueberries, bananas and oranges
- veggie sticks: carrots, celery, sugar snap peas, broccoli, cauliflower and lettuce wraps
- stew with rice packed on top to keep the stew together and warm
- sushi (sushi rice recipe)
- gluten-free pretzels with grain mustard dip
- raw nuts/seeds and dried fruit
- yoghurt with fruit, fat-free Greek yoghurt, etc.
- red pepper strips with tzatziki
- taco salads/nachos: chips, guacamole/avocado, salsa, shredded lettuce, shredded chicken
- chicken or tuna salad
- risotto with seasonal vegetables and/or seafood
- hummus with veg sticks, pitta, rice cakes or corn crackers.

Tea

Baking a good gluten-free cake is a technical challenge, whether at home or commercially. Cakes and biscuits without gluten can too easily be dry, heavy, gritty and highly unappealing. Successful products require careful experimentation with a mix of ingredients such as gluten-free flours (e.g. rice or maize flour), possibly along with starches, fibres and the latest addition that helps add sticky chewiness – Xanthan gum, which is a stretchy starch with characteristics similar to gluten.

'Together, I find these can work well in baking,' says Angela Mumby of Food Ambitions, one of a growing band of food technologists who are making their mark by discovering alternatives to baking with gluten.

Whether you invest in one of the many gluten-free cook books now available or buy shop-made cakes, there's no reason at all to go without. Large bakeries such as United Central Bakeries in Edinburgh and Bells of Lazenby near Penrith have developed hugely popular ranges of cakes and biscuits. One of the fastest-selling free-from cakes in the UK is Mrs Crimble's award-winning chocolate macaroons, which – say the manufacturers – is successfully targeted at consumers generally.

Dinner

Dining at home should not pose a problem for those with gluten intolerance. There are 195,000 edible plants in the world. Yet on average, in the West, we get 50 per cent of our calories from wheat, points out nutritionist Anthony Haynes.

It's worth bearing in mind that the majority of the world's population never consume gluten. Meat or fish along with root and green vegetables with fruit are naturally gluten free. In Italy, which is responsible for some of the world's most delicious gluten-containing foods, notably pasta and pizza, there are large geographical areas where pasta and bread are never eaten – where the staple is polenta, made with maize meal.

It's also worth recalling the Paleolithic diet at dinnertime. Our hunter gatherer forefathers ate a naturally gluten-free diet, including everything that isn't made by man: meat, fish and seafood, fruits and vegetables, as well as nuts and seeds.

Of course, you may find that gluten-free or gluten-light alternatives to gluten-containing food come into their own, to add variety to what is a potentially unsatisfying and monotonous menu. If that's the case, then you don't need to worry that what you're eating is unhealthy – gluten-free alternatives to pastas and pizza are no more unhealthy than the real thing.

Researchers at Hammersmith Hospital investigated concerns that the gluten-free alternatives had a higher glycaemic load than gluten-containing foods. The glycaemic load is the amount by which your blood sugar increases during the two hours after you eat. Food with a low glycaemic load, and therefore a low measure on the glycaemic index, is known to be healthier because it causes fewer sudden changes or spikes in blood sugar levels.

But there was no cause for alarm. The researchers from the hospital's Department of Nutrition & Dietetics reported online in 2002 that there was no difference between the glycaemic index of gluten-free and gluten-containing foods, and therefore no extra risk of health for people with gluten intolerance.

Even so, it's worth bearing in mind that there are far more nutritious alternatives to pasta and pizza, such as teff, quinoa, millet, buckwheat and brown rice. Diet experts also recommend this low glycaemic load approach to gluten-free eating as the best way to keep off unwanted weight.

Louise, 39

'Free-from food is expensive and not really worthwhile. After all, you can eat everyday food that doesn't have any gluten in it. I might sometimes buy corn pasta or something like that. But mostly, dinners for me are rice and potato based, with lots of salads with some grilled chicken or fish. One of my favourite dishes is stewed lentils with rice and vegetables like leeks and courgettes. It's really satisfying and delicious, and something I would never have thought of eating before I went on a gluten-free diet. A gluten-free diet certainly works for me all right. I cut 15 minutes off my marathon time without doing any extra training.'

9

Living gluten free

Identifying the problem is just the first step to managing gluten intolerance. You can't have surgery or put yourself on a course of drugs to cure this health problem. You have to live the treatment every day. A gluten-free diet is difficult but increasingly do-able, and all the more so if you are aware of and prepare for the pitfalls ahead. Here are some key strategies to make sure that you don't give up on living gluten free.

Make sure you get a proper diagnosis

If you think you have got coeliac disease, it's important to get a diagnosis. To do this successfully, it's essential to continue to eat gluten until investigations are done to make a definite diagnosis. This is because taking gluten out of the diet, or reducing the amount of gluten eaten before being tested, is likely to cause false-negative tests.

If you've already cut gluten out of your diet, then you will need to reintroduce it to ensure that the tests for coeliac disease are meaningful. Deciding to be tested for coeliac disease may involve making a conscious effort to include more gluten-containing foods in your diet. Coeliac UK (see Useful addresses, at the end of this book) recommends that you eat the equivalent of four 'servings' of gluten-containing foods for a minimum of six weeks before you are tested. A serving of gluten might be a slice of bread, a portion of wheat-based cereal, two digestive biscuits or four tablespoons of pasta.

Once you have a diagnosis, you will have access to free prescription gluten-free staple foods and food ingredients, including bread, flour, bread mixes and pasta. You will also be eligible to join Coeliac UK, which is a uniquely supportive charity where membership is restricted to those with a diagnosis of coeliac disease.

As well as campaigning and funding research, the organization provides expert and independent information to help people manage their health and diet – with a diet and health helpline, a food and drink directory, an Eating Out Without guide, as well as a regular magazine and a recipe database. It also has local support groups throughout the UK.

If you have non-coeliac gluten intolerance, a diagnosis is just as important. It's quite possible to get a diagnosis with a variety of methods, of which the gold standard is the exclusion diet. This is best carried out with the help of a health practitioner.

Expect a gluten reaction

Stopping any type of food can cause withdrawal symptoms, and gluten is no exception. Expect your symptoms to get worse before they get better. Withdrawal symptoms may seem to be exactly the same as those caused by the intolerance itself, with common reactions including diarrhoea, abdominal bloating and cramping, joint pain, anxiety, depression, clumsiness, fatigue, shortness of breath, rapid pulse, mouth ulceration, muscle cramps or twitches, insomnia, restless legs, weepiness, irritability, constipation, irritable bowel symptoms, feeling hopeless, itchy skin rashes, generalized itching that travels around the body and headaches. The above symptoms normally last for a couple of days, but they can last for several days or even weeks.

You may also experience cravings for gluten-containing food. All of this will fade if you persist with the diet. Try to focus every day on what you can eat rather than on what you can't.

Expect an emotional gluten reaction

Change is difficult at any time, and having to change your diet and cut out food that you're used to and enjoy eating can be frightening, depressing and isolating. Remember that it's normal to feel angry and frustrated at the lack of choice that you feel you are facing, and that you, and only you, are having to cope with this hardship. You're in shock and having to cope with change – this is not a permanent emotional state. Most people can and do adapt to a life of gluten-free dietary fulfilment.

Exercise is a good coping mechanism

Going to the gym, starting to jog or run, or even going for walks in the fresh air will raise your mood and get your brain producing mood-enhancing endorphins.

Exercise programmes that are designed to get rid of unnecessary tension can also be helpful. These include yoga, tai chi and simple breathing exercise as well as Pilates and Alexander technique.

A course of lessons in Alexander technique can be particularly helpful. By learning how to move with less effort, you should find that you will free up more energy and take the pressure off your joints and organs, including your digestive system. Well-being is enhanced, and alongside improved breathing and organ function, you are likely to have better digestion and absorption of nutrients.

Resist the temptation to cheat

Face up to your moments of weakness, whether it's the desire to fit in with others, or that as it's a special occasion, it's just this once and shouldn't matter. It's all too easy to slip from an imposed discipline. You may consider you have the preceding valid reasons to go gluten just this once, but each time you may be making it more difficult to follow a gluten-free diet.

Keep an eye on your health

You need to be aware of the health problems that you may have to face in the future, even if you keep to a strict gluten-free diet. There are two different ways in which your health might be affected by gluten intolerance. First, the physical characteristics that have made you vulnerable to gluten intolerance may also make you vulnerable to other disorders. Second, the experience of having unrecognized gluten intolerance, possibly for several years, will have had an impact on your physical health. For both of these reasons, you should alert your GP to your diagnosis and make sure you have access to the right health screening and medical care.

Associated conditions

Other autoimmune diseases

Coeliac disease is an autoimmune disease that appears in people who have the genes that predispose them to develop it. For this reason, people with coeliac disease are more likely to develop other autoimmune diseases, such as type I diabetes and thyroid disease.

Lactose intolerance

This seems to be associated with gluten intolerance and the symptoms are similar. They include nausea, bloating, abdominal pain and diarrhoea. When the lining of the gut is damaged by active coeliac disease or by gluten intolerance, the body may not make enough lactase. Lactase is the enzyme that the body normally produces to help break down the lactose, a sugar found in milk from cows, sheep and goats, but not in soya or rice milk.

Once the gut is healed after a few months of being on a gluten-free diet, lactose intolerance should no longer be a problem. But in the early months, it may make sense to cut out all dairy products, particularly if the symptoms of coeliac disease seem to be persistent.

If you are avoiding dairy products, it's important to make sure that you find alternative sources of calcium. Among the best sources are green vegetables, such as broccoli and kale, and fish with soft, edible bones, such as salmon and sardines.

Serious complications

If you have had long-standing, poorly controlled gluten intolerance, then you are likely to be more at risk of osteoporosis or osteopenia, though this will be minimized by following a gluten-free diet.

- Osteoporosis is a condition in which the body's bones become brittle and more likely to break. It's diagnosed by measuring bone mineral density (BMD), which assesses the strength of bones. Osteopenia describes a BMD that is lower than normal, but not as severely so as in osteoporosis. People who develop or are diagnosed with gluten intolerance later in life could be at greater risk of developing these disabling disorders. Engage in weight-bearing exercise such as walking, jogging and gardening. It's even more important than ever to stop smoking. You should also talk to your GP to see whether it's worth getting a referral for a bone health test, known as a dual energy X-ray absorptiometry (DEXA) scan, which measures your BMD.
- You could also have a small risk of lymphoma of the small intestine – a problem that until recently was considered a major issue for people diagnosed with coeliac disease, but which has now been shown to be rare. Research has shown that the risk among people with coeliac disease is no greater than for anybody else after three to five years on a gluten-free diet.

Remember you can still get digestive problems

Once you have the symptoms of gluten intolerance under control, it can be tempting to consider the problem to be solved for life. It isn't necessarily so. A stomach bug can still damage your digestive system, and your symptoms are likely to return if you don't follow a strict gluten-free diet.

Julia
When Julia was diagnosed with coeliac disease, she followed a strict gluten-wheat free diet and began to feel much better. Just 18 months later, however, she got a stomach bug. 'I was in New York at the time and no-one seemed to know anything about gluten-free shops or cafés. And all hell broke loose. It was as if I had started from scratch with terrible stomach pains and horrible diarrhoea. I could hardly stand up at one point. It was so depressing. I just didn't feel I could start all over again. Thank goodness I was able to access support from people who log on to a support group. They were able to help me in a way that people who were physically close to me couldn't. I don't know what I'd do without them.'

Pay attention to detail in the kitchen

Keep gluten-free kitchenware free from gluten

Unless you live in a household where everyone eats gluten-free food, you'll need to take special measures in order to be able to follow a strict gluten-free diet. These include the following:

- keeping separate cooking utensils – you could colour code them with tape to help you keep track of spatulas, wooden spoons, bread and cutting boards, and even pans if it speeds up cooking;
- using separate toaster, microwave and perhaps even separate shelves in the fridge and freezer;
- treating breadcrumbs and other gluten-containing remains as a source of contamination, at least as bad as bacteria – get rid of them;

- check medicines to make sure they are gluten free – most are but there is a chance that you may be prescribed older pills that contain gluten.

John and Debbie (parents of Janet)
'When our daughter, Janet, went to university, we had to buy her her own fridge freezer, microwave and toaster so that her food wouldn't be contaminated by non-gluten-free products. Once we knew we had to do it, it was straightforward. But it just didn't occur to any of us, until right at the last minute.'

Start baking

You might as well accept one single unhappy fact – gluten is an all but essential ingredient of decent-tasting bread. As Andrew Whitley points out in his classic book Bread Matters (see Further reading, at the end of this book), 'Wheat gluten is unique. You can't mimic it except by using strange additives that aren't food.' So gluten-free bread is rarely a success. And the closer it gets to real bread, the more unhealthy it seems to be. Gluten-free bakers tend to use 'all the chemical contrivances in the book to create something that displays as many of the characteristics of standard white wheat bread as possible, including: soft squishy texture, a bland flavour and above all, "a significant dose of artificial additives".'

So what do you do? The obvious answer is to turn your back on bread. Corn tortilla wraps are a great alternative to sandwiches, for instance. Gluten-free muesli is a good alternative to wheat-based cereal, and you can eat potatoes or rice instead of pasta or pies.

If you want to bake your own bread, Whitley's excellent advice is 'not to mourn the absence of gluten but to relish the qualities of flours that do not contain it'. His recipes include combinations of different types of flour: corn, chestnut, gram and manioc to make yeasted gluten-free bread; and brown rice flour, corn, buckwheat and manioc to make rice, brazil nut and linseed bread.

If you are going to bake your own bread regularly, you can save time by mixing up large quantities of your favourite gluten-free flour mix and then storing it and weighing out the quantities you need. There are also some excellent bread mixes made from combination flours.

Other types of gluten-containing foods have proved much easier to mimic. Commercially produced gluten-free cakes and biscuits have a much better reputation than bread. Top quality brands such as Mrs Crimble are actually beginning to compete with non-gluten-free brands. And it's becoming relatively common to find cake recipes in magazines that actually call for gluten-free ingredients because they work better for that particular taste.

Karen, 43
Gluten hides itself in a lot of products, so it makes sense to stop buying processed foods. I tend to make everything like bread from scratch. I don't buy from supermarkets because they're a lot more expensive than normal foods, and you can make them yourself. I've lost the sense of what wheat-based products used to taste like, and I'm used to the loss.'

10

Shopping gluten free

Eating well on a gluten-free diet used to be regarded as difficult, if not impossible. 'It was a question of: Well, what can we eat?' recalls Michelle Berriedale Johnson who founded the magazine and website Foods Matter in 2000. The answer, she says, was 'Not a lot.'

Gluten-free food was widely acknowledged to be 'fairly disgusting' – stuck in a 'food as medicine' rut, with little incentive or interest in improvements. 'After all, you're ill and therefore the NHS doesn't think you should have anything enjoyable,' commented one GP, describing the gluten-free fare that is still available on prescription for anyone with a diagnosis of coeliac disease.

In just a decade, however, all that changed. 'Today, if something doesn't taste that nice or isn't nicely presented, it won't survive – because there'll always be something that tastes nicer and looks better,' says Michelle.

Sales of gluten-free food in larger supermarkets and online are soaring as never before, with manufacturers investing in finding alternatives to gluten-containing cereal and new ways to make gluten-free food taste good.

Shopping online makes sense when you're buying gluten-free products regularly. Gluten-free food is exactly the kind of niche market that has flourished on the internet – enabling scores of small companies, many of them starting off with just a handful of products, to find sufficient customers to allow them to expand significantly.

There are now a number of well designed websites that target people with food intolerances while providing a highly professional online service. They supply useful information about each product, such as what it contains and whether it can be frozen, and the purchase can be completed in minutes. What's more, next day mailing, which is now routinely reliable, makes internet shopping thoroughly sensible.

At the same time, larger supermarkets today stock wide ranges of gluten-free foods. You can buy branded and own brand pot noodles and bean burgers, vegetarian pates and frozen ready meals as well as gluten-free sausages, fish fingers and chicken nuggets – with gluten-free trifle or tiramisu for afters. There are endless mixes for gluten-free bread, baguettes and pitta bread rolls as well as gluten-free pasta and pizza bases, and even a gluten-free version of Coco Pops.

But it is gluten-free cakes and biscuits that have proved the great success of gluten-free products. The arrival of the gluten-free Jaffa Cake in 2002 was a cause for celebration in families with gluten-intolerant youngsters. 'It was a really good day and made the whole family feel better,' recalls Sheila Large, 43, who has two daughters with coeliac disease. 'For the first time, my girls could have a treat that their friends took for granted. They felt that bit more normal, and my other two children were also pleased because they were able to have Jaffa Cakes again.'

Since then, gluten-free cakes and biscuits have just got better and better. Bells of Lazenby's apricot and cinnamon range of cakes and Mrs Crimbles' range of cakes are targeted and enjoyed by a wide range of customers beyond the gluten intolerance market. As such, they are identified in what market researchers described in 2008 as a new trend – the 'not so naughty but still nice' foods that are healthy and delicious.

Here are three ways to make sure that you get the best gluten-free products from the supermarket.

Be selective

Remember, as with everything else, the quality varies, and with gluten-free products the worst can still be fairly bad. So be prepared to try a few varieties before you give up, and check out what other people think.

Coeliac UK (see Useful addresses, at the end of this book) produce their annual Food and Drink Directory that lists several major supermarkets' own branded products, and it is free to members. Foods Matter is an organization devoted to taste as well as food intolerance. The findings of their regular tastings, published on their website <http://www.foodsmatter.com>, are informed and detailed, making the website and the magazine a must read for anyone with a food intolerance.

The scope of Foods Matter

To give an idea of the scope of Foods Matter, in a single month in 2008 the Foods Matter team judged 'excellent' gluten-free pate (<http://www.britishfinefoods.com>) and 'extremely appealing' fun gluten-free pastas for kids (<http://www.funfoods4all.com>), as well as the following gluten-free foods:

- Conscious Foods (India) nibbles, including cashew, coconut and walnut nugget, sesame chews (<http://www.consciousfoods.co.uk>), with 'exotic and wonderful flavours, all delicious and amazingly healthy';
- Chris Thompson's Seed Stacked Flapjacks made from honey, oats, sesame, sunflower, linseed and pumpkin, 'and seriously delicious' (<http://www.seedstacked.co.uk>);
- EnerG's gluten-free doughnuts (<http://www.GeneralDietary.com>), 'a somewhat surprising colour but very good – rather solider than a conventional doughnut, they are still quite spongy with a pleasant, slightly fruity flavour'; and
- gluten-free Asda milk chocolate wafer bars (<http://www.asda.com>) – 'unassuming little bars that bear a strong resemblance to Aero-filled KitKat, containing milk, egg and soya as well as rice, potato and teff flour'.

It's not just the big websites that can be helpful. Lots of people with gluten intolerance write their own blogs, with their own strong opinions and genuine experience of shopping gluten free. There are also websites that provide chat room space, where people with food intolerance can swap ideas and tips, and frequently their good and bad experiences of gluten-free food shopping.

Keep checking the label

When Raf, 32, was diagnosed with gluten intolerance in 2005, it was the need to check labels that caused the most irritation. 'I want the labelling to be absolutely trustworthy and obvious at a glance so that I don't have to check through the small print scanning the ingredients. If I had nut allergy, I would get that. With gluten, I mostly don't.'

Such irritation is understandable. All pre-packaged foods in the UK are covered by current European Commission (EC) legislation, which requires manufacturers to identify ingredients containing gluten. This means that if a gluten-containing cereal (wheat, rye, barley, oats or spelt) is used as an ingredient, it must appear on the ingredients' list, regardless of the amount used. At the moment, however, there is no requirement to include an advice box that says 'Contains gluten', although this is recommended.

This causes problems, largely because of inconsistencies. Most crisp manufacturers today, for instance, are aware of the issues for people with gluten intolerance and make it absolutely clear whether a packet of crisps contains gluten or not (some don't). In 2007, a new rice-flavoured crisp came onto the market, which only listed wheat starch as an ingredient in the small print. In fact, wheat starch was the major component of the rice-flavoured nibble, albeit with most, but not all, of the gluten removed. The rice, so visibly apparent on the packaging, made up only 26 per cent of the product. As such, the crisp was toxic at least for people with coeliac disease, although possibly acceptable for those with gluten intolerance.

Until 2012, when new legislation is due to be introduced to deal with the problem of labelling, it is essential that anyone following a gluten-free diet check both the list of ingredients as well as the 'allergy advice' box. In other words, even if the packaging says 'gluten free', you can't necessarily rely on it.

Different manufacturers also use different symbols and words to mean gluten free. Coeliac UK's Crossed Grain Symbol is widely used to show that the food is approved by the charity. But some supermarkets use their own version of the Crossed Grain Symbol, and the words in the advice box vary between manufacturers. They may say

- 'gluten free'
- 'suitable for coeliacs' or
- 'suitable for a gluten-free diet'.

As yet there is no specified difference in meaning in all of these phrases, and certainly no uniformity throughout the EC. It's hardly surprising that people with gluten intolerance find shopping a time-consuming toil.

Even the term 'gluten free' is not clear. It's generally used to indicate a harmless level of gluten rather than a complete absence, something that is difficult to achieve except in naturally gluten-free food such as rump steak or tangerines.

The exact level at which gluten is harmless is uncertain and controversial. A recent systematic review tentatively concluded that consumption of less than 10 milligrams of gluten per day is unlikely to cause an abnormal response, though the truth is that very few reliable studies had been done.

New EC legislation on food labelling, passed in July 2008, is the first attempt for decades to clarify all this. And although it will not be enforced until 2012, it is likely that the vast majority of food manufacturers will begin to introduce the new rules from 2009.

The new labelling system follows the standard for gluten-free labelling, set by an international body called Codex Alimentarius, a body within the World Health Organization. It is this standard-setting body that sets the level of gluten permitted in gluten-free products, and this has recently been updated providing – for the first time – a dual standard, with two categories of gluten-free foods.

- *'Gluten free': foods containing less that 20 ppm (parts per million) gluten.* In the future, only foods that contain less than 20 ppm can be labelled 'gluten free'. This will apply to specialist substitute gluten-free products, such as breads containing wheat codex starch with less than 20 ppm. It will also include naturally gluten-free mainstream products like soups, beans and crisps. Pure, uncontaminated oat products with a gluten level of less than 20 ppm may also be labelled gluten free.
- *'Very low gluten': foods containing between 20 and 100 ppm gluten.* Products containing gluten above 20 and up to 100 ppm will be labelled 'very low gluten'. This will particularly apply to specialist substitute gluten-free products (such as breads and flour mixes) that contain codex wheat starch, a specially processed wheat starch that has a level of gluten within the Codex standard.

There are other improvements in labelling that some companies are already scrupulously providing, and which are likely to spread throughout the industry, even though not covered by legislation. You have a right to expect a high standard of information on products, including through the manufacturers' websites. Cadburys, for instance, carry a list of their products on the front page of their website, showing what allergens are contained in each one. You should also expect clear labelling when products contain gluten where it is not expected, such as in wheat sugar, an ingredient that is widely used in convenience foods.

Accept the price of gluten free is likely to be higher than normal food

Gluten-free food is considerably more expensive than their gluten-containing equivalents, costing up to five times as much, when compared with a supermarket's own brand food. The cheapest own brand white bread or packet of pasta is around 35p. The gluten-free equivalent is £2.50 or more. It's a cause of concern for many people, according to Coeliac UK.

Yet a visit to a commercial gluten-free baker quickly reveals why the cost of gluten-free food is more than gluten-containing foods. Bells of Lazenby supplies gluten-free cakes, biscuits and bread to all of the leading supermarkets, including Asda, Booths, Boots, Morrison's, Sainsbury's and Waitrose, as well as Cumbrian Co-op stores and local shops throughout the North West. Its success is built on considerable investment. Back in 2002, it established links with Manchester Metropolitan University Department of Food Science to carry out research to underpin their product development. The company was awarded a Department of Trade and Industry Smart grant for research and development activity, and then made a significant investment in building a dedicated bakery to create a new brand, OK, alongside its established Village Bakery. It then employed the sales expertise to get the product to market – winning a Queen's Award for its efforts.

Whereas many producers operate in mixed environments where flour ingredients are used alongside their 'free-from' counterparts, Bells has insisted on the highest standards from their suppliers and tests finished products to the lowest attainable levels that can be tested for in externally verified laboratory conditions. Companies such as Bells are the ones that are currently flourishing and look likely to continue to do so.

Naturally gluten free

As always, people with gluten intolerance can safely buy a whole range of foods that are naturally gluten free, many of which are extremely nutritious. The list includes all fresh fruit, vegetables, meat, fish, nuts, herbs and spices, as well as the following:

- vegetable and olive oils, mayonnaise and salad dressings
- frozen fruits and vegetables, plain canned fruits and vegetables, tinned beans and lentils
- tinned tuna, salmon and sardines
- milk, cream, whipping cream, sour cream, butter, margarine, yoghurts and cheese, including cottage and cream cheese
- eggs, tofu, rice pudding and tapioca pudding
- rice cakes, rice crackers, corn tortillas and popcorn
- dried fruit
- chocolates
- organic packaged soups
- anything made from quinoa, rice, buckwheat, chickpeas, flax, sunflower seeds, cornstarch or potato starch
- vinegar, mustard, ketchup, horseradish, jams, honey, relish, pickles and olives
- cornflakes and rice krispies
- sugar, salt and pepper
- cornmeal, baking soda and baking powder and
- coffee, tea, soft drinks, 100 per cent fruit juice.

Avoid
It is probably wise to assume that anything pre-wrapped or processed is best avoided, as it may include gluten-containing additives.

Gill, 28
'I buy gluten-free crackers, corncakes, rice cakes, cakes and biscuits, and pizza bases. Sainsbury's is very good and they do frozen gluten-free food.'

Louise, 39
'Watch out on cosmetics. Some lip balms and lipsticks contain gluten.'

Will, 34

'After several months of following a gluten-free diet, I finally found cakes that taste nice. They are Caramel Shortcake slices made by SunStart. So far I have had them from Asda and Tesco. I have also found that Asda's fruit cake slices are lovely! I am a fan of fruit cake, and was gutted when I thought I could never have Christmas cake again!'

James, 23

'I've found gluten-free crisps (Walkers), popcorn and Snack a Jacks. I'm hooked on Haribo Starmix, which is fine, and Lees do a gluten-free snowball and macaroons.'

11

Going out and staying gluten free

You can be well organized and self-sufficient when you are at home, but in the big wide world you are reliant on other people – and, too often, that can mean being at the mercy of their prejudices about gluten intolerance.

Attitudes to food intolerance are clearly changing – you only have to walk through a supermarket to realize that. But it's worth bearing in mind that considerable confusion about food intolerance remains, particularly among those who pride themselves on their guts and their ability to consume and digest whatever is put in front of them.

'Where were all the coeliacs when we were kids? Where were those battalions of people who couldn't eat bread or pasta because it made their tummies hurt?' asks respected restaurant critic and wit Jay Rayner in his weekly *The Guardian* column in November 2007. He goes on in similar vein, deciding that they probably weren't 'locked up in their parents' attic' or 'chained to the radiator, just waiting for the moment when the *Daily Mail* would recognise their plight in a double page spread, providing employment to quack nutritionists so that they could suddenly walk among us nibbling their bloody rice cakes and looking all puppy-eyed and self-pitying.'

Rayner has a sharp-tongued wit that is frequently directed against restaurateurs – and this, alongside his excellent judgement, is the reason for his unparalleled reputation as a food columnist. But calling people with coeliac disease and other food intolerances 'attention-seeking frauds', and as grown-up versions of 'the tiresome little brats who, as children, spat out everything put their way with a shout of "I don't like it"' takes sharp-tongued wit to another level. The fact that it remains on the *The Guardian* website (at least until publication of this book) shows just how fun and cool it is to be intolerant of food intolerance.

As was pointed out in the deluge of protests at the time, such criticism is grossly unscientific. Yet anyone with a food intolerance is likely to have come across such an attitude, especially if they attempt to eat out at a café, restaurant or hotel. In far too many cases, staff are not just ignorant about gluten intolerance, but they can also be irritated by customers who are too often seen as making extra trouble for busy chefs.

Once again, however, things are changing. Here's a guide to getting the most out of gluten-free eating outside the home.

Tim, 42

'Eating out is such a predictable nightmare. I have to check that something looks gluten free on the menu before asking staff to check that it is in fact gluten free: Theatre Royal in Plymouth – please take note that couscous is made from wheat. Coping with the stress has brought my relationship to breaking point more than once.'

Raf, 32

'My moments of relapse usually occur when I'm eating out. On my last birthday, for instance, I was given a gift voucher for an expensive restaurant that doesn't cater for gluten intolerants. I suffered for several days afterward, had terrible bowels for nearly a week but I can't say I regret it.'

Emma, 29

'I've got so used to being treated as a nuisance whenever I eat out. It's amazing to suddenly find places that cater for gluten free. I came across a tea place a few months ago that served gluten-free scones and suddenly there are lots of them. I even found a tapas chain that actually seems to welcome people with gluten intolerance – and suddenly Spanish food is my favourite.'

Eating out gluten free

If you are gluten intolerant, you will know how hard it is to eat safely away from home. From top-class restaurants to the local chip shop, awareness of how to cater gluten free is generally poor. A recent survey of 3000 people with coeliac disease revealed that more than 58 per cent felt that eating establishments do not offer clear gluten-free options, and 59 per cent don't trust staff to know enough about preparing gluten-free food.

Yet eating out is possible with a little forethought, enabling you to enjoy your life rather than staying stuck at home. For a start, there is growing pressure on the catering industry to look after people with gluten intolerance, as they already have taken account of vegetarians and people with peanut allergy.

'The lack of information in restaurants and other catering outlets is a major source of frustration for coeliacs, who are far less likely to eat out as a result,' points out Sarah Sleet, Chief Executive of Coeliac UK (see Useful addresses, at the end of this book), launching the charity's year long Food Without Fear campaign in January 2008. With seven out of ten of its members saying that they have virtually given up eating out, the charity wants to turn around what it sees as a serious problem. 'It is time for the catering industry to wake up and realise that there is a substantial niche market that they are missing out on.'

In another initiative, Coeliac UK teamed up with the National Trust between February and May 2009 for a 'Free for Tea' campaign, with several of the Trust's cafés and restaurants serving gluten-free options at least for the duration of the campaign.

A sign of the times was an episode of the popular 2008 BBC2 series *The Restaurant*, during which contestants in the competition – judged by Raymond Blanc – had to cater for customers with special diets. These included vegans and vegetarians, but also real people with gluten intolerance. The vegans ended up with cabbage and not much else in one case. And the competitive restaurateurs inevitably attempted to serve non-gluten-free options to the customer with gluten intolerance – who, fortunately, questioned everything they were concerned about. But the point was made. When summing up, Raymond Blanc was adamant about the importance of ensuring that all special diet customers are well served.

Coeliac UK has also backed an excellent initiative Gluten-Free on the go (<http://www.gluten-free-onthego.com>), a website set up to help people with gluten intolerance to find hotels, restaurants and cafés that cater for those requiring a gluten-free diet, as well as helping caterers contact suppliers and even advertisers of gluten-free products. There are places to eat throughout the UK as well as in France, Italy, Spain and Majorca.

All of the venues listed on the website have signed up to the Gluten-Free on the go code of practice, which covers all aspects of food service:

- ingredients
- storage
- preparation techniques
- avoidance of cross-contamination
- training and taking customer service for those with gluten intolerance seriously.

This initiative is also being underpinned by new EC legislation due to come into force in 2012 that will require caterers to provide detailed food labelling for customers relating to allergy and intolerance, including gluten intolerance.

Restaurant chains that serve gluten-free food are also listed on I'm Gluten Free Baby (<http://www.imglutenfreebaby.co.uk>), a delightful gluten-free blog, largely devoted to gluten-free recipes, written by blogger Cat, who is 'a full on foodie who loves cooking, eating out and holding dinner parties. The thing is I'm on a gluten free diet, and it's hard loving food so much when it doesn't love you back.'

Cat recommends the following:

- Wagamama (<http://www.wagamama.com>), which guarantees two gluten-free meals on its nationwide menu;
- Nandos (<http://www.nandos.co.uk>), which has gluten-free chicken, rice, coleslaw and sweetcorn, but NOT chips;
- ASK (<http://www.askrestaurants.com>), a chain of Italian restaurants that has several gluten-free sauces and guarantees that it will cook gluten-free pasta if you bring it.

She also gives justifiable publicity to the Angel Inn near Sheffield, where gluten-free beer is permanently on tap and there is an entirely gluten-free menu every Tuesday (0114 289 0336).

It all shows what's possible, and suggests the way forward. In the meantime, here are three ways to get the best service if you've got no choice but to eat at a restaurant you don't yet know.

- Phone beforehand to ask whether they cater for special diets. If they ask what gluten is, then you should probably try a different venue. It's also worth asking whether all of the food is prepared on site, and whether a recipe can be tailored specially for you.
- When you arrive at the restaurant, check the menu and ask to talk to the chef. You need to mention the important factors, including the need to use different chopping boards and cooking utensils for preparing gluten-free food. Don't go into too much detail – just mention the important facts.
- After the meal, be sure to say 'thank you' for the care and attention you have been given. Remember that whatever the chef learned from the experience will only help the next person who asks, 'What do you have that is gluten free?'

Of course, once you have found somewhere that looks after you, the chances are you will visit again. And don't forget to let fellow coeliac sufferers know where they can eat safely.

Go on a gluten-free cookery course

Learn how to avoid cross-contamination and gluten-free cooking times and temperatures at one of a new type of cookery course, targeted at those embarking on a gluten-free diet. Sarah Garwood of Newlyns Cookery School, Hook, Hampshire, offers an evening demonstration of how to create gluten-free alternatives to classic dishes (<http://www.newlyns-farmshop.co.uk>)

Find a gluten-free partner

Include the fact that you're gluten intolerant if you're trying out internet dating. If you are looking for someone to date, or to start a new relationship, possibly with someone who shares your need for a gluten-free diet, then add your profile to the site, and in addition to your other interests include the words 'gluten free' or 'coeliac'.

Religious ceremonies

Most mainline Christian churches offer their communicants gluten-free alternatives to the sacramental bread, usually in the form of a rice-based cracker or gluten-free bread. These include United Methodist, Christian Reformed, Episcopal, Lutheran, The Church of Jesus Christ of Latter-day Saints and many others.

There's a problem for Catholics with gluten intolerance, however. Roman Catholic doctrine states that for a valid Eucharist the bread must be made from wheat. Requests for permission to use rice wafers have always been denied. However, a low-gluten host was approved for use in Italian masses in 2002 and two years later in North American services, with each host made and packaged by hand in a dedicated wheat-free, gluten-free environment.

There has also been a long-standing discussion on the question of the ordination of priests with gluten intolerance. On 22 August 1994, the Congregation for the Doctrine of the Faith apparently barred people suffering from gluten intolerance from ordination, stating, 'Given the centrality of the celebration of the Eucharist in the life of the priest, candidates for the priesthood who are affected by coeliac disease or suffer from alcoholism or similar conditions may not be admitted to holy orders.'

After considerable debate, the congregation softened the ruling marginally in 2003. 'Given the centrality of the celebration of the Eucharist in the life of a priest, one must proceed with great caution before admitting to Holy Orders those candidates unable to ingest gluten or alcohol without serious harm,' it said.

Jewish law holds that a person should not seriously endanger one's health in order to fulfil a commandment. Thus, a person with severe gluten intolerance is not required, or even allowed, to eat matzo – unleavened bread made in a strictly controlled manner from wheat, barley, spelt, oats or rye – at the Jewish festival of Pesach (Passover). In any case, many kosher Passover products avoid grains altogether and are therefore gluten free.

Packed lunches

Peter Thomson can still remember the bread he had to eat when he took packed lunches to school when he was first diagnosed with coeliac disease several years ago. 'It came in a cylindrical tin and I could only describe the taste as a mixture between cardboard and polystyrene! I had to drink copious amounts of water to get it down.'

Packed lunches, revolving as they do around sandwiches made from only slightly improved gluten-free bread, can still be a problem. Yet they are, if anything, more important for people with gluten intolerance. Too often, schools still regard a request for a gluten-free diet as an example of 'difficult' or picky behaviour. At work, access to a microwave or kitchen area to prepare and heat food may cause concerns about the risk of contamination. And while some airlines manage to provide gluten-free alternatives without fuss, many passengers with gluten intolerance have to put up with food that isn't gluten free or at best put up with soggy rice cakes and a salad.

Here are five ideas from Peter Thomson listed on his website (<http://www.peter-thomson.co.uk/glutenfree>) to use leftovers in the most delicious way to beat the packed lunch blues, and spread the cost of a gluten-free diet.

- Meals that were served hot the night before can be eaten cold for lunch the next day.
- For hot meals and home-made soup, try using a vacuum flask. Put the food in the refrigerator overnight and then reheat before leaving for work or sending the children off to school.
- Buying a slightly larger joint of meat for the Sunday roast can leave plenty to make Monday's lunch.
- Cook extra rice, potatoes or pasta the night before; these can be the basis for many easy gluten-free recipes.
- Use chopped, leftover boiled potatoes, other cold leftover vegetables such as peas, halved cherry tomatoes, canned sweetcorn (corn on the cob), cheese cubes, chopped raw mushrooms, sultanas, chopped apple and anything else you can find. Just pop all of the ingredients into a plastic lunchbox and mix in a little gluten-free mayonnaise or salad cream. Season well and enjoy!
- Fresh fruit, of course, also makes a healthy finish to any

packed lunch. An apple or banana or even a small bunch of grapes can be tucked into your lunchbox. Or make a gluten-free sponge pudding and save a piece to pop into your lunchbox the following day.

Useful addresses

Allergy UK
3 White Oak Square
London Road
Swanley
Kent BR8 7AG
Allergy Helpline: 01322 619898
Website: www.allergyuk.org

The operational name of the British Allergy Foundation, a leading charity in the field of allergies and intolerances of all kinds. Fact sheets and articles are published, and the latest information is available on a wide range of conditions, including gluten intolerance.

British Nutrition Foundation
High Holborn House
52–54 High Holborn
London WC1V 6RQ
Tel.: 020 7404 6504
Website: www.nutrition.org.uk

Provides information, through publications, educational resources and conferences, on healthy eating and the relationship between diet, physical activity and health, based on the interpretation of scientifically based knowledge.

Coeliac UK (formerly the Coeliac Society)
Suites A–D, Octagon Court
High Wycombe
Bucks HP11 2HS
Tel.: 01494 437278
Helpline: 0870 444 8804
Website: www.coeliac.org.uk

The leading charity working for people with coeliac disease, with a mission to improve the lives of people living with the condition, through support, campaigning and research. It provides expert and independent information to help people manage their health and diet, campaigns to improve access to fast diagnosis and good subsequent healthcare and safe foods, as well as researching new treatments and the possibilities of a cure. Anyone who has been medically diagnosed with coeliac disease can join the charity.

www.foodreactions.org
Set up by Dr Mario Cassar, formerly a biochemist in the NHS, specifically targeting people with food intolerance. It has a lively forum and also sells enzymes for treating food intolerance.

Foods Matter
5 Lawn Road
London NW3 2XS
Tel.: 020 7722 2866
Website: www.foodsmatter.com

An organization that publishes the results of its regular tastings of gluten-free food, holds an annual Foods Matter Free From Foods Awards, and publishes the UK's only magazine supporting anyone living with allergies or on a 'free-from' diet. Their website is a forum for members and also a well-organized archive of articles and research on allergy and food intolerance.

Online access to advice and gluten-free food

www.gluten-free-onthego.com
Provides an easy way to look for a hotel, restaurant or café to manage your gluten-free diet. Listed venues have been recommended by visitors who have an understanding of gluten intolerance.

www.glutenfree.wordpress.com
Inspirational blog by the American amateur chef and coeliac, Kate Chan.

Harmony Cuisine
www.harmonycuisine.co.uk
A new online resource set up by Paul and Emer Mander-O'Beirne after Emer developed Crohn's disease and found difficulty getting hold of credible, reliable and easy to understand nutritional information on what foods improve or worsen different medical conditions. For a small monthly fee, members have access to a team of expert dieticians, chefs and home economists providing clinically researched information on nutrition as well as individually tailored recipes.

www.imglutenfreebaby.co.uk
A blog largely devoted to gluten-free recipes, written by Cat, 'a full on foodie who loves cooking, eating out and holding dinner parties. The things is I'm on a gluten-free diet, and it's hard loving food so much when it doesn't love you back.'

www.innovative-solutions.org.uk
A website providing details of buying teff flour (a kind of flour made from grains that do not contain gluten).

www.peter-thomson.co.uk/glutenfree
Peter Thomson's website giving recipe advice and providing a forum for people with gluten intolerance.

Advisory websites

www.bda.uk.com
The website of the British Dietetic Association – the professional association for registered dieticians in the UK. As such, this organization represents the only nutrition professionals to be statutorily regulated, and governed by an ethical code, to ensure that they always work to the highest standard. Dieticians work in the NHS, private practice, industry, education, research, sport, media, public relations, publishing and organizations both governmental and non-governmental. Their advice influences food and health policy across the spectrum from government, local communities and individuals.

www.fabflour.co.uk
This website produced by the Flour Advisory Bureau promotes the role of bread and flour as part of a balanced diet. Among other informational items given are details of gluten-free grains, and a recipe database.

www.icak.com
The website of the International College of Applied Kinesiology, a system that evaluates structural, chemical and mental aspects of health using manual muscle testing with other standard methods of diagnosis.

www.mind.org.uk/foodandmood
The Food and Mood Project, the web-based user-led company providing dietary self-help resources for improving mental and emotional health, closed in January 2009 and its website <www.foodandmood.org> was taken over by the national mental-health charity Mind.

www.stat.org.uk
The website of the Society of Teachers of the Alexander Technique, which uses physical and psychological principles to co-ordinate the body, often resulting in the relief of muscular pain.

Shows and exhibitions

The Allergy and Gluten Free Show: **www.allergyshow.co.uk**
Foods Matter Awards: **www.freefromfoodawards.co.uk**

Bakeries and shops

Artisan Bread Original (ABO)
Tel.: 01227 771881 (Mondays and Thursdays)
Website: www.artisanbread-abo.com

A mail-order enterprise run in Whitstable by Tom and Ingrid Greenfield, who make organic rice-flour bread, using natural leaven and a seaweed-based flavour enhancer instead of salt.

Bells of Lazonby
Edenholme Bakery
Lazonby
Penrith
Cumbria CA10 1BG
Tel.: 01768 898437
Website: www.ok-foods.co.uk

An award-winning family bakery which stocks an innovative range of gluten-, wheat- and dairy-free foods. They supply Booths stores throughout the north of England and other shops, including supermarkets, throughout the UK.

Drossa Ltd
Tel.: 020 7431 9382
Website: www.drossa.co.uk

This company sells gluten-free products from around the world, with a guarantee that 'just because it's gluten-free doesn't mean it's flavour free'.

The Gluten Free Kitchen
Tel.: 01969 666999
Website: www.theglutenfreekitchen.co.uk

A dedicated bakery producing gluten-, wheat- and dairy-free cakes, puddings and savouries that are also free from additives and preservatives. Their coffee and walnut cake won an award in the Foods Matter Gluten Free Awards 2008 category of gluten-free cakes, muffins and puddings. Sales are largely through the thriving mail-order facility or online, but the website also provides information on where their products may be bought, and also lists restaurants and other outlets where they are available.
For outlets throughout Ireland, contact Juniper Fine Foods (01387 249333).

Infinity Foods
25 North Road
Brighton BN1 1YA
Tel.: 01273 603563
Website: www.infinityfoods.co.uk

This shop was set up as a workers' co-operative in 1971. Selling wheat-free flour and other whole and vegetarian foods, it is open from 9.30 a.m. to 6 p.m., Monday to Saturday.

Mrs Crimbles
Tel.: 08451 300869
Website: www.mrscrimbles.com

Established during the 1980s, this company provides cakes and biscuits that are free from wheat, gluten and dairy ingredients. It claims its products are made to the highest standard, and they can be found in all good independent farm shops, health stores and delicatessens. Nowadays they are also to be found in the 'free from' or speciality sections of the more well known supermarkets.

Newbury Phillips
Website: www.newburyphillips.co.uk

Their gluten-free naan and pitta breads are available from As Nature Intended stores in London (phone 020 8840 4856) and in Hale, Greater Manchester (phone 0161 928 1719).

Roley's
Website: www.roleys.com

A small bakery based in the Netherlands which combines traditional artisan skills with the use of special natural 'rediscovered' ingredients to produce high-quality innovative products that are now available in the UK. Their Teff Flour Mix was awarded the Best Free From Food Product Trophy 2008 by the Foundation for Allergy Information and Research. Their products are available from Sainsbury's, Somerfield, Waitrose and Asda supermarkets as well as many wholefood stores nationwide.

It should be noted also that most major supermarkets offer wide ranges of special-diet foods and advisory leaflets, and extra information is available on their websites.

The Village Bakery
www.village-bakery.com

A pioneering organic bakery and brand established just over 30 years ago by Andrew Whitley (see also the site www.breadmatters.com). They use natural processes, artisan methods, renewable energy and interesting ingredients to make their organic and special dietary foods (including gluten-free ranges), supplying supermarkets throughout the UK.

Further reading

Brostoff, Professor Jonathan and Challacombe, Stephen J., *Food Allergy and Intolerance*. Burlington, MA, Saunders, 2002. (This is the principal medical textbook on the subject.)

Brostoff, Professor Jonathan and Gamlin, Linda, *The Complete Guide to Food Allergy and Intolerance*. London, Bloomsbury Publishing, third edition 1998.

Groves, Barry, *Trick and Treat: How healthy eating is making us ill*. London, Hammersmith Press, 2008.

Hunter, Dr John, Workman, Elizabeth and Woolner, Jenny, *Solve Your Food Intolerance*. London, Vermilion, revised edition 2005.

Thomson, Peter, *Gluten-Free Cookery: The complete guide for gluten-free or wheat-free diets* (Beginners' Guides). London, Hodder-Arnold, revised edition 2001.

Whitley, Andrew, *Bread Matters: The state of modern bread and a definitive guide to baking your own*. London, Fourth Estate, 2006.

Index